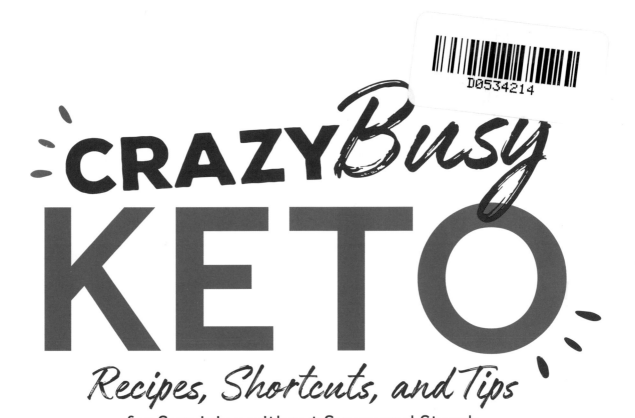

# CRAZY Busy KETO

## Recipes, Shortcuts, and Tips

### for Surviving without Sugar and Starch

## Kristie H. Sullivan, PhD

Victory Belt Publishing Inc.

Las Vegas

*This book is dedicated to my sweet family, who have endured a crazy busy mom who, as they truthfully describe, never cooks anymore because she's too busy writing cookbooks!*

*It is because of you three that I am both crazy and busy. I love you more than bacon.*

First published in 2019 by Victory Belt Publishing Inc.

ISBN-13: 978-1-628603-92-7

Cover design by Crizalie Olimpo
Front cover photo by Hayley Mason and Bill Staley
Interior design and illustrations by Kat Lannom and Charisse Reyes

Printed in Canada
TC 0119

# Contents

# WHO ISN'T CRAZY *Busy?*

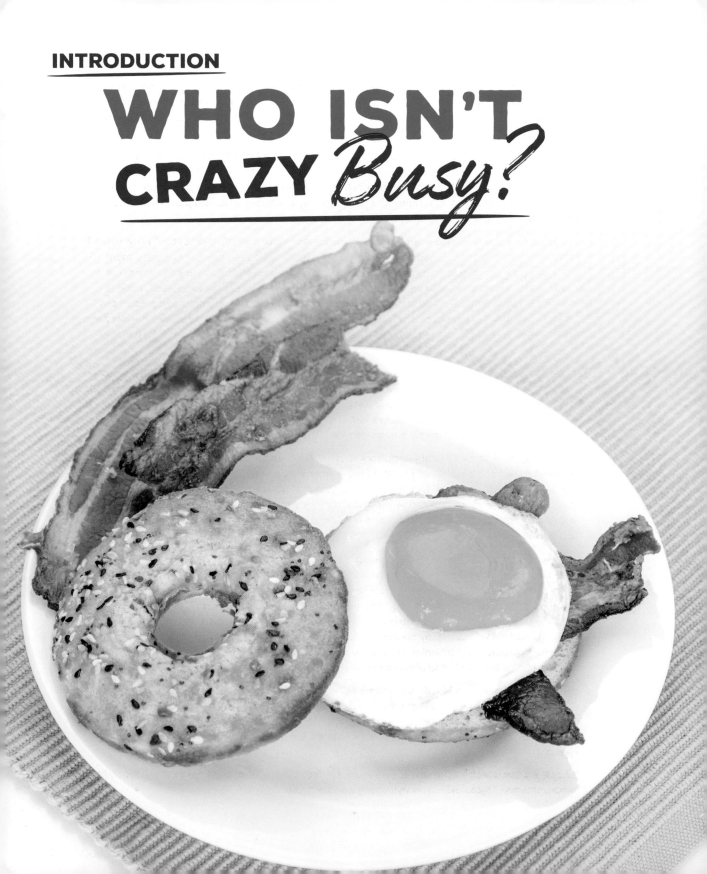

I started a ketogenic diet just after my kids' school year ended in June 2013. Summer is usually less hectic for my family because there's no homework, no extracurricular activities, and a lazier agenda for the kids. Even though I was in the middle of a huge project at work, I knew that summer was a better time than fall to begin to create new habits.

In fact, our lives have never *not* been crazy busy. Before keto, I had found a few time-saving tips that had helped me survive working full-time, finishing a PhD, wrangling toddlers, and commuting to work and school. I recognized that I needed to use some of those same strategies to make keto work. If I didn't, I knew that this new way of eating would fall apart when school began and life became *really* crazy busy.

Looking back, my life only became *more* busy after that work project ended. I continued to work full-time, created a social media presence, and wrote three books while surviving as a mom with two kids going from elementary school through middle school and into high school and doing every extracurricular activity known to man! Did I mention that I also served as a PTA officer for two years and volunteered at church and with other community and school organizations? And my husband works out of town, so I am the taxi driver, appointment scheduler, and primary contact for everything related to the kids, including doctors and specialists. And I love every minute of it!

Not only have our lives been hectic, but we've had the typical challenges of crazy busy families—medical emergencies with extended family members, hospital stays, extended and unexpected travel, last-minute schedule changes, storms that brought power outages, and holidays that bring the best kinds of crazy stress. In short, we've found ways to make keto work all day, every day, even under the most hectic circumstances.

My friends and extended family know that I have a laundry basket yardstick for how busy we are. If the eight laundry baskets we own are empty and the hampers aren't overflowing, then life is under control and serene. If the laundry is washed and folded and waiting in the baskets to be put away, then we're busy but managing with minimal stress. If the kids are getting dressed from clean clothes tossed unfolded into four different baskets and a clean load of laundry left in the dryer, then it's desperate times indeed.

I imagine you have your own way of assessing when you're merely busy versus crazy busy and feeling as if you're just barely holding everything together. This book is here to help you get through those crazy busy times without setting aside your healthy keto lifestyle because it's "too hard" or "too time-consuming." The recipes in this book include simple meal ideas, easy recipes that require minimal or no cooking, and more difficult recipes that can be prepped in advance so that you can enjoy great meals even when there's little time. I've also provided tips for incorporating convenience foods to make meals with excellent keto macros as well as strategies for sticking to the plan when traveling or when you only have access to a microwave.

This book was designed for all those times when life isn't perfect, but when it's real, like when the laundry baskets are running over with clean but unfolded laundry. When "perfect" eating might have to take a backseat to "good enough." My grandmother called it giving life "a lick and a promise," meaning that you keep trying by taking a lick at it and promise to do better when you can.

I hope you can use the tips and recipes in this book to take a good lick at being consistently keto with a promise to yourself to always prioritize your health.

# MANAGING KETO While CRAZY Busy and STAYING SANE

How do I do it? How do I keep my on-the-go family of four, with differing picky preferences, eating keto while managing to stay reasonably sane? This section outlines some of my best strategies for making keto manageable with minimal advance planning.

## GENERAL TIME-SAVING TIPS AND HACKS

### HAVE A GENERAL PLAN.

You don't have to meal plan, but you should know what easy keto meals can be made quickly and keep the ingredients for those meals stocked in your kitchen. See my shopping lists on pages 12 to 16 for help determining which foods to keep on hand.

### KEEP IT SIMPLE.

When dishes are easy to make, they become the ones that we enjoy repeatedly. One meat or other protein source and one vegetable is perfect. Or choose one- or two-dish meals that make cleanup even easier, such as my Double Bacon Cheeseburger Bake (page 52), Easy Chicken and Beef Enchilada Bake (page 78), Shrimp Salad–Stuffed Avocado Boats (page 82), or Quick Chicken Chowder (page 90).

Another way to simplify your life is to try recipes that require minimal cooking, such as my Spicy Poppin' Shrimp (page 100), or no cooking whatsoever, such as my Buffalo Chicken Ranch No-tato Salad (page 50), Chipotle Chicken Salad (page 68), Cold Tossed Pizza Bowl (page 74), or Thai Chicken Slaw with Peanut Sauce (page 84). Another tactic is to choose recipes that can be made in the microwave, like the Lemon Minute Muffins (page 32).

If you're looking for something even simpler to keep you keto at the busiest of times, check out the easy ideas for breakfasts, main meals, super fast sides, and snacks at the beginning of each recipe chapter.

## COOK SMART!

When you're already in the kitchen dirtying pots and pans, you might as well make the best use of your time. I do so in a few ways.

First, I like to "cook double." My cooktop has five burners, and I can generally keep an eye on two or three burners at a time. While I brown ground beef for taco salad, for example, I can also cook quarter-pound hamburgers for a meal later in the week. I might have two skillets to wash afterward, but if the dishpan is already full of hot soapy water, then I save time by not washing the skillet later in the week.

One of my best breakfast survival tips is to bake a frittata while eating dinner on Sunday evening. By the time dinner is over and the kitchen has been cleaned, the frittata is baked and cooled. It can then be sliced and refrigerated for quick, nutritious breakfasts on hectic weekday mornings.

You can also cook double by doubling recipes and freezing portions for later. An inexpensive set of freezer-safe glass or plastic food storage containers makes it easy to freeze individual portions that can be warmed on demand.

Second, I prep ingredients for future meals while making a meal. For example, with the cutting board out, I can easily chop multiple vegetables. While I might use only one onion at a time, my future self is thankful to reach into the fridge and grab an already-diced onion for a meal later in the week. Bell peppers, broccoli, cauliflower, and celery are other great veggies to prep in bulk. You can also toss those extra diced veggies into a stir-fry, an omelet, or a frittata to make a meal in no time.

Lastly, I like to use my slow cooker to cook meats such as whole chickens and turkey breasts, and even for browning ground beef. I season the raw meat in the morning and set the slow cooker to low for eight hours. When I come home, dinner is mostly ready to serve.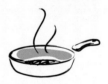

## CLEAR THE CLUTTER.

You really don't need a ton of kitchen appliances or gadgets to successfully follow keto. Don't tell my husband, since I really love appliances and gadgets, but the following equipment is more than enough:

- a good set of knives
- a cutting board
- one or two trusty skillets
- a small and a medium-sized saucepan
- a few microwave and oven-safe glass containers in varying sizes
- a set of cooking utensils that includes tongs

Keeping the clutter down in the kitchen helps me feel less stressed and gives me more room to prep and cook meals.

Having said that, a food processor, a slow cooker, a silicone baking mat, and a spiral slicer can make life in the kitchen much easier.

## INVEST IN A GLASS FOOD STORAGE CONTAINER SET.

I recommend glass food storage containers such as those made by Pyrex or Anchor Hocking because they save a lot of time and effort in the kitchen. You can bake or microwave in them. You can also use them as serving dishes. Any leftovers can be stored quickly using the lids that come with them, and leftovers can be reheated in the same container. I've even been known to eat directly from the container when there is only a single portion left over.

## USE CONVENIENCE FOODS AND PRODUCTS, INCLUDING SHELF-STABLE ITEMS.

Sometimes perfection is the enemy of "good enough." Yes, it is wise to pay attention to ingredients, but be creative, especially when traveling. You might be surprised at where you can find the ingredients for a simple meal to keep you going.

Use grocery store convenience items, for example. Even grocers in rural areas often have food bars or salad bars. One of our local stores has a breakfast bar with sausages, eggs, and *bacon!* The bacon is crisp and warm and waiting every morning. You can put as much or as little as you like in a carryout container. Because it doesn't weigh very much, buying precooked bacon is a true bargain in terms of money and time, especially when you don't have to clean a skillet or baking pan afterward. The only downside is that you don't get to capture the rendered bacon fat for cooking.

Grocery store food bars also tend to have chicken wings. We buy them plain without sauce and season them ourselves with our favorite seasonings, like Chili-Lime, Greek, and Traditional Buffalo (all on pages 70 to 73).

One of my favorite hacks is to use the salad bar to make a meal that isn't a salad. Salad bars often feature protein sources such as chopped hard-boiled eggs, ham, pepperoni, and bacon. In addition, the vegetables are cleaned and already cut into bite-sized pieces. When a recipe calls for a small amount of a meat or vegetable or a wide variety of vegetables, buying only what you need from the salad bar can save you time and money.

I've included a couple of my favorite salad bar meals in this book: the Salad Bar Crustless Quiche on page 38 and the Salad Bar Stir-Fry on page 96.

See page 12 for meal ideas using shelf-stable foods. Also, refer to the section "Keto Outside of Your Kitchen" for a list of items that should be easy to find while on the go.

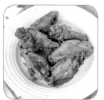

**Chili-Lime Wings**
*page 70*

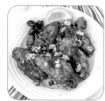

**Greek Wings**
*page 72*

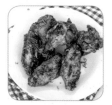

**Traditional Buffalo Wings**
*page 73*

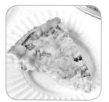

**Salad Bar Crustless Quiche**
*page 38*

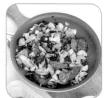

**Salad Bar Stir-Fry**
*page 96*

*Kristie Sullivan*

## HAVE A PLAN B (AND A PLAN C, D, E...).

One of my favorite sayings is, "You always need a plan, and then make a Plan B." In fact, on many days I need a Plan C, D, and E so I don't get an F for the day!

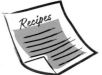

When my children were very young and I was commuting in opposite directions to work and graduate school and dragging them along to daycare or elementary school, I had a list of what I called Plan B meals. These were meals that I could make quickly and could pull together from ingredients I always kept stocked in my fridge, freezer, or pantry. Before keto, they included a lot of convenience foods, such as frozen waffles, frozen chicken tenders, frozen lasagna, spaghetti sauce, pasta, rice, canned veggies, and canned fruit or fruit cups. We ate microwaveable meals and lots of packaged products such as cereals, crackers, and granola bars.

When we went keto, my challenge was to transition from a menu of highly processed high-carb convenience foods that we all enjoyed to low-carb, high-fat alternatives that could be made equally quickly and were equally tasty and convenient. I reasoned that if I could have ten high-carb Plan B meals, then I could also figure out ten keto Plan B meals. Just as I needed those meal options to survive on a standard diet, I needed options to survive, and thrive, on keto.

I started by brainstorming everything quick that my family enjoyed, knowing that most of what I pulled from the freezer would need to be foods I had prepared and frozen in advance. Here are fifteen of our favorite Plan B options that you may want to try:

1. **Cooked burgers**—As mentioned earlier, sometimes I cook burgers while I'm making something else for dinner on Sunday evening. We can eat the burgers for lunch or dinner during the week, or I can freeze them for later. To warm them, I take them from the fridge or freezer and put them in a skillet with a lid. I add a few tablespoons of water and heat them until they are warmed. Then I remove the lid, brown them up, and serve them with mayonnaise, bacon, cheese, avocado, and other keto-friendly toppings. These are especially nice to have on hand when we're all eating on different schedules.

2. **5-Minute Lasagna**—All the ingredients for this recipe are always in my fridge or freezer. Save time by freezing precooked ground beef or Italian sausage in single-serving packets along with the cheese. Not only can the kids make this dish for themselves, but they feel like they are getting a first-rate meal. The recipe is on page 54.

3. **Rotisserie chicken**—I can run into the grocery store and grab a rotisserie chicken faster than I can go to a drive-thru. Grab a bagged salad from the produce section and you have a ready-made meal. Plus, you can make chicken salad with any leftover meat.

4. **Chicken, ham, tuna, or shrimp salad**—Canned meats are shelf-stable and ready whenever you need them. I keep a variety stocked in the pantry for making quick meals. You can prepare a basic chicken salad with mayonnaise, hard-boiled eggs, dill pickles, salt, and pepper. I've also included a quick shrimp salad recipe on page 82, which you can stuff into avocado boats or eat on its own. These are great options for lunch boxes or an easy dinner.

5. **Egg salad**—You can make it from eggs that are purchased boiled or boil your own. Egg salad is a great lunch option as well as an easy dinner that will keep when the family is eating on different schedules. There's an Easy Egg and Bacon Salad recipe on page 92.

6. **Meat sauce**—Ground beef takes about ten minutes to brown, and I always have jarred spaghetti sauce or canned tomato products and spices on hand. My family eats meat sauce over zoodles, konjac noodles, or spaghetti squash (see page 122)—or even with a spoon as long as there is plenty of cheese sprinkled over the top.

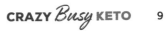

7. **Pan-seared steak**—All it takes is high heat, some bacon fat, and ten minutes from fridge to table for a medium-rare steak. Dinner doesn't get more simple or delicious than this! My quick recipe is on page 94. Even though a steak needs no side, bagged salad or Loaded Baked Yellow Squash (page 122) makes it a full meal.

8. **Taco salad**—This can be made with leftover chicken, ground beef, or steak; you can even season the cooked meat in advance and freeze it for later. When you pull the seasoned meat from the freezer, warming it in a skillet or the microwave takes only a few minutes. You can pile the meat onto romaine lettuce (a head of romaine lettuce tends to have a longer shelf life than other lettuces or packaged prewashed lettuce), a bed of pork rinds, or store-bought Parmesan chips. Top it with cheese, sour cream, or jarred salsa for a quick and tasty meal. If you're lucky, you'll have a perfectly ripe avocado to add to your plate.

9. **Meatballs**—Just like burgers, I make an effort to have some cooked meatballs stored in a freezer-safe bag. They can be tossed into tomato sauce to simmer until warmed through, or they can be added to a lunch box frozen. They won't be warm by lunch, but they will be thawed and ready to eat. One of our favorite versions is the Greek Meatballs on page 88.

10. **Deli meat wraps**—More than once, my children have made a meal out of deli meat wrapped around cheese sticks. It's a lunch staple that can be dipped in mayo, ranch dressing, or another fatty sauce. We buy canned olives and single-serving packs of dill pickles to add extra flavor.

11. **Bacon and eggs**—Not just for breakfast, and super easy to make if you use precooked bacon. We buy several packages of warehouse club–sized precooked bacon (think Costco or Sam's Club) each month. Even my twelve-year-old can warm up some bacon in a pan and then scramble some eggs in the bacon fat without assistance.

12. **Shortcut Pizza Crusts**—These are ideal for my family because we all enjoy different pizza toppings. Prebaked individual crusts can be taken from the freezer, placed on a baking sheet, topped, baked, and served in less than thirty minutes. You can also cook these pizzas in an air fryer in about ten minutes. The recipe is on page 56.

13. **Pulled pork BBQ**—Sometimes I freeze leftover pork when my husband smokes a pork shoulder. Other times I freeze pulled pork purchased by the pound from local restaurants. Either way, you have a quick meal just by adding some low-carb BBQ sauce and a serving of canned or frozen green beans. If there's time, you can make a quick coleslaw using bagged cabbage.

14. **Cold Tossed Pizza Bowl**—This Plan B meal uses pepperoni and fresh mozzarella cheese and is even better the day after it's made. Another kid favorite, this dish is great for lunches and for travel. Find the recipe on page 74.

15. **Waffles**—Just as we did in the old high-carb days, we can have waffles on the go. I make them ahead of time and refrigerate or freeze them. They can be toasted just like store-bought waffles and used to make breakfast sandwiches that the kids can finish eating in the school car line awaiting drop-off. The recipe is on page 42.

Use these fifteen ideas to help get you started creating your own list of Plan B meals. We rotate these meals so that we don't become bored with them. We may not love them every time we eat them, but we know that we are well fed and on plan, and that's what matters most.

Don't forget that restaurant meals can be great Plan B options, too. See the Crazy Busy Restaurant Guide on pages 20 to 22 for suggestions.

## COMMUNICATE YOUR FOOD PLAN TO OTHERS IN YOUR HOUSEHOLD.

Nothing derails a meal plan like someone using up an ingredient or eating something I need to make a meal. And I generally don't discover that the item is missing until I'm rushing to make dinner. That's why I started creating a simple list that I post on the fridge. The first part includes my plan for the week's meals. It reminds me to get all the ingredients at the store or to make sure I have what I need in the pantry or freezer. At least one night a week, I plan for leftovers. The list looks something like this:

## Dinner

| | |
|---|---|
| **MONDAY** | Fried Salmon Patties with Creamy Cucumber and Red Onion Salad |
| **TUESDAY** | Greek Meatballs with Tzatziki Sauce |
| **WEDNESDAY** | Salad Bar Stir-Fry |
| **THURSDAY** | Leftovers |
| **FRIDAY** | One-Pan Chicken Alfredo with Spaghetti Squash |
| **SATURDAY** | Dinner out |

The second part of the list includes foods that I've prepped ahead of time or leftovers that anyone can grab for breakfast or lunch. It also includes foods that need to be used up, such as avocado or deli meat. I began doing this when I noticed that I was tossing things because we'd simply forgotten they were there. My husband was buying lunches out when I was throwing away foods that he would have enjoyed. Keeping this list taped to the fridge is an easy way to remind him, and me, of what is readily available. It also keeps the kids from whining, "Mom, there's nothing to eat!" when in fact there is!

Throughout the week, we cross off an item when we've eaten the last of it, and I add items that are left over from prior meals.

## To Eat!

| | | |
|---|---|---|
| Everything Bagels | ~~Chipotle Chicken Salad~~ | Avocado |
| Good Morning Granola | 5-Minute Lasagna | Chili-Lime Trail Mix |
| | ~~Deli meat~~ | Peanut Butter Fudge |
| | Greek Meatballs with Tzatziki Sauce | |

## BE YOU.

Spend time thinking realistically about what works for your family. If you don't like canned chicken, don't buy it. If you want to eat scrambled eggs seven days a week, then eat them! The challenge for many of us is not to strive for lofty ideals like those that bombard us on social media, but to develop practical strategies that become automatic and allow us to make the most of our limited time.

# STAYING STOCKED

As you might have guessed, my crazy busy meals work because I keep my kitchen well stocked, especially the freezer and pantry, where foods tend to wait for me a bit longer than they do in the fridge. In this section, you'll find lists of the items I like to have on hand.

## PANTRY STAPLES FOR QUICK MEALS

These pantry staples may not be perfectly perfect, but they are excellent choices for pulling together quick meals when life gets crazy busy. Canned meats like tuna can be made into salads, added to a bed of fresh greens with a nice fatty dressing, or used in a stir-fry. I've used canned meats to make several of the casseroles in this book; see the notes that accompany the recipes. You can also use jarred or canned veggies to complete a meal and/or to add flavor and use fats to increase satiety and to keep your meals keto—quickly, easily, and tastily!

| COOKED MEATS AND PROTEINS (IN PACKAGES, JARS, OR CANS) | LOW-CARB VEGGIES (IN JARS OR CANS) | FATS |
|---|---|---|
| bacon | artichoke hearts | avocado oil |
| chicken | chipotle peppers | coconut oil |
| crab meat | collard greens | ghee |
| ground beef | diced tomatoes (plain and with green chilies) | mayonnaise |
| pulled pork | green beans | olive oil |
| sardines | jalapeño peppers | sesame oil |
| shrimp | olives | tallow |
| tuna | pickles | |
| nut and seed butters (almond, peanut, etc.) | roasted red peppers | |

*Kristie Sullivan*

## SHELF-STABLE BASICS

The following is a list of shelf-stable basics that you will want to keep stocked for a variety of purposes. For example, instant coffee powder can be used in very small amounts to add depth to chocolate recipes or even gravies and sauces.

- alternative sweeteners*
- baking chocolate (unsweetened)
- broth (beef and chicken)
- cocoa powder (unsweetened)
- dark chocolate (90% cacao or higher)
- instant coffee powder

- sea salt (fine-grained)
- vanilla extract
- vinegar (apple cider, balsamic, and white)
- whey protein isolate**

> *Crazy Busy Kitchen Tip:* Mix vinegar with avocado oil or olive oil to make a quick salad dressing or a marinade for less expensive cuts of meat.

### *A note about sweeteners

My preferred sweeteners are the products made by Sukrin USA, which include a blend of stevia and erythritol as well as a monk fruit blend. I detect no aftertaste when I use these sweeteners, although some others do. I use these products when sharing foods with others and find that most people enjoy foods made with the Sukrin blends.

Please be aware that the goal of using alternative sweeteners is to have minimal impact on blood glucose. If you are diabetic, you should always test to see whether a particular sweetener affects your blood sugar. In general, the three safest options are stevia, erythritol, and monk fruit, with the caveat that those who are allergic to ragweed may experience an allergic reaction to stevia. Also, erythritol may cause stomach upset in some people, although it is less likely to be problematic than other sugar alcohols.

### **A note about whey protein isolate

Whey protein isolate is the only form of whey protein that I use, and I use it solely for baking. The protein provides structure to baked goods in the absence of gluten. Whey protein isolate has nearly all the lactose (milk sugar) and casein (milk protein) removed. My preferred brands, Isopure and Jay Robb, have zero carbs and are made from reasonably good ingredients.

If you can't use whey protein isolate because you avoid dairy, you can try substituting an equal amount of unflavored egg white protein powder. Be sure to read the ingredients and use a brand with zero carbs. Jay Robb is a good brand to try.

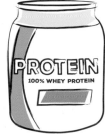

## CONVENIENCE SAUCES

These convenience sauces can be used to make super quick meals when paired with a protein. While they may not be as good as homemade sauces, they do not have to be made, which saves time. My favorite brands are listed in the Shopping Guide at the back of the book.

- béarnaise
- chimichurri
- enchilada sauce
- hollandaise
- pesto

## DRIED SPICES

Just six basic spices can liven up your meals without taking up a lot of space in your pantry or breaking your grocery budget. If you have these essential seasonings on hand, you can make nearly anything taste good!

- black pepper
- chili powder
- garlic powder
- ground cumin
- Italian seasoning
- onion powder

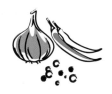

# FRESH AND FROZEN FOODS FOR QUICK MEALS

## REFRIGERATED ITEMS

For the fridge, there are certain items that I almost always buy. In fact, if any of the following items are on sale, I check the use-by date and buy two or three packages at a time. I've never had to throw out butter or cream! In fact, I'm often grateful to find that last package lurking in the back of the fridge.

- bacon
- breakfast sausage
- butter (I use both salted and unsalted)
- charcuterie
- cheese, including full-fat mozzarella, Parmesan, cheddar, fresh mozzarella
- cream cheese

- deli meat
- eggs (large size for use in recipes)
- heavy cream
- Italian sausage
- pepperoni
- sour cream

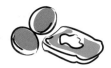

*Kristie Sullivan*

## FRESH MEATS

Fresh meats have a shorter shelf life than many of the basics listed above, so I don't buy a lot of them at once; however, if I find my preferred fatty cuts on sale, I buy them for the freezer. Having two or three packages of meat in the fridge at the beginning of the week typically guarantees at least a few good meals for the family. Steaks in particular are super quick to cook without feeling rushed.

- beef ribs
- chicken thighs (with skin)
- chicken wings
- chuck eye steaks
- ground beef
- pork ribs
- pork steaks
- rib-eye steaks
- salmon
- shellfish (cleaned)

## FRIENDLY VEGGIES

When it comes to veggies, fresh ones are my first pick, but produce isn't always forgiving if you forget it for a day or two. When it comes to the best low-carb options, I tend to think of veggies as "friendly" or "unfriendly." Friendly veggies are like dear old friends whom you might not see often, but when you do see them, you can pick right up where you left off. Friendly veggies have a reasonably long shelf life and will wait a little longer for you to remember them than other vegetables—or there are good canned or frozen options available.

As for unfriendly veggies, I view them as unforgiving. They refuse to be forgotten for more than a day or two. They won't wait for you when you're a day late on your meal plan. They go bad before you're ready for them. Like an unreliable partner, they aren't always there when you need them.

Failing to consider shelf life is a common mistake. Wasting food and money makes me feel bad. It also leaves me with fewer options for meals. There's nothing worse than opening the fridge and finding that the fresh salad you were planning to eat left "fresh" behind a few days ago. Friendly veggies know that I sometimes have visions of freshly made meals that get interrupted by lost credit cards, emergency vet visits, or children yelling, "Mom! I need you!" Friendly veggies wait their turn longer. While they can expire, too, friendly veggies have more patience for a hectic lifestyle.

These are a few of my favorite veggie friends that are low-carb and reliable. Many are also available frozen or canned.

- bell peppers
- broccoli
- Brussels sprouts
- cabbage
- cauliflower
- celery
- jalapeño peppers
- onions
- zucchini

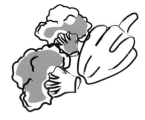

## NOT-SO-FRIENDLY VEGGIES

These veggies are not so friendly when fresh but are good frozen or canned:

- asparagus
- avocados
- green beans
- kale
- mushrooms
- spinach

While I do buy unfriendly veggies, I try to buy them when I know I'll have time to cook or eat them soon. I can't help but love the low-carb value of lettuces, fresh herbs, and cucumbers. They are not as friendly, but they are delicious! Never turn your back on an unfriendly veggie. It will turn brown on you before you can say "crazy busy." If you're particularly busy, stick with the friendlier veggies that are also your low-carb favorites.

## FROZEN ITEMS

The freezer is a handy tool. Just like the pantry, most items will wait for you in the freezer. Here are a few basics that I keep stocked:

- bacon
- ground beef
- meats that I find on sale, such as chuck roasts, whole chickens, pork tenderloins, and pork shoulders
- sausage
- shredded cheese
- veggies such as broccoli, riced cauliflower, green beans, and spinach

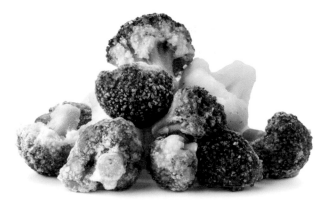

*Kristie Sullivan*

# KETO OUTSIDE OF YOUR KITCHEN: BUSINESS TRAVEL, VACATION, CAMPING, ETC.

My life is often busiest when I'm on the road, even if I am traveling for vacation. I've found that regardless of the reason for travel, the keys to success are packing good shelf-stable options, finding effective strategies for keeping foods cool, and knowing what to look for when buying foods away from home.

## SHELF-STABLE FOOD OPTIONS

Perhaps one of the biggest struggles when trying to follow a ketogenic diet on a busy schedule is the lack of good shelf-stable options. Highly processed foods that are also high in refined carbohydrates are shelf-stable and convenient. They can last for months on pantry shelves and survive in purses, lunch boxes, suitcases, desk drawers, and camp duffels.

Instead of old standbys such as granola bars and boxed cereals, keto requires that we have good sources of protein and fat, which can be tricky when eating on the run. That's why I've put together this list of shelf-stable keto staples that are ideal for travel, camping, and other on-the-go activities. Ideal packages of these foods are those that contain just one serving.

- coconut oil packets
- Epic bars (Check the ingredients; not all flavors are keto-friendly.)
- ghee packets
- jerky (Check ingredients and nutritional information; some brands have as many as 6 to 8 grams of carbs per serving. Look for those with less than 2 grams per serving.)
- mayonnaise packets
- mustard packets
- nut butter packets
- olive cups or packs
- pepperoni pouches
- pickle packs
- pork rinds
- precooked bacon strips or pieces
- ranch dressing packets
- sardines (in flip-top cans)
- tuna pouches

## STRATEGIES FOR KEEPING FOODS COOL WITHOUT A COOLER

While many hotels provide small in-room refrigerators, I find myself without refrigeration from time to time when I'm traveling. When that happens, I use a few hacks to keep small items like butter, cheese, and heavy cream cool.

- **Large cup**—Most convenience stores have huge Styrofoam cups for fountain sodas and will charge you a quarter or less for a cup. I usually fill it half full with ice, and then I can put small food items in the ice.

- **Ice bucket**—Even if hotels don't have mini refrigerators, they often have ice machines and ice buckets. I use the plastic liners to hold ice and keep smaller items cool.

- **Large and small freezer bags**—Freezer bags make great travel companions. A gallon-sized bag can hold ice from a convenience store or a hotel ice machine. A smaller pint- or quart-sized bag can also hold ice or keep foods dry as the surrounding ice melts.

## WHAT TO BUY AND WHERE TO BUY IT WHEN YOU'RE ON THE MOVE

More than once, I've left home without a cooler or a bag of groceries. Unless you're traveling to a Third World country, you can almost always find something acceptable to eat, even if it isn't ideal. Whether I'm traveling for business or for pleasure, I often rely on grocery stores, convenience stores, and/or discount stores, which may be among the few options available to you in rural areas.

### GROCERY STORES

My favorite source for foods while traveling is grocery stores. You can easily buy a few key items to make several inexpensive meals without stopping at a restaurant.

In addition to using the salad bar or hot food bar for obvious choices, such as chicken wings and grilled meats, check out the deli counter. You will likely find a variety of meats and cheeses, along with ready-to-eat offerings like chicken salad and chef salads. The specialty meats and cheeses section often has a variety of charcuterie and sliced cheeses for ready-made tapas. When traveling, I look for locally sourced cheeses that I might not find closer to home. I sometimes splurge on Burrata (cream-filled fresh mozzarella) and salami, soppressata, or prosciutto, which tastes like a gourmet meal in any setting.

Don't overlook the platters that are designed for entertaining. Many are great options for lunches because the meats and cheeses are sealed in individual pouches. I've found trays with three different meats and cheeses that provide three satisfying meals for less than $10. Another option is prosciutto- or pepperoni-wrapped mozzarella, which has great protein and fat.

While I don't often buy fruits or veggies while on the go, I might buy fresh berries as a treat. For additional fat or flavor, you can also find olives, pickles, salad dressings in individual packs, premade guacamole, or a fresh avocado, which comes perfectly packaged for travel.

Lastly, grocery stores obviously carry shelf-stable products such as nuts and nut butters, as well as butter and heavy cream for coffee. See page 12 for shelf-stable ideas.

## CONVENIENCE AND DISCOUNT STORES

Here are some items that I've found at convenience stores and even dollar stores while on the go, even in rural areas. Again, not all of these foods are ideal—some are highly processed—but if you have limited options, a can of Spam is better than a package of saltines.

- beef jerky
- canned tuna
- cheese (string cheese or cheddar)
- condiment packets—mayonnaise, mustard, hot sauce
- hard-boiled eggs
- hot dogs or sausages without the bun
- nuts—almonds, cashews, peanuts, or mixed nuts
- packaged sandwiches with the bread discarded
- pork rinds
- potted meat or Spam
- sardines
- Vienna sausages

Stores like Dollar General and Dollar Tree tend to have even more options than those listed above. In particular, I've found a wide range of canned meats that provide excellent protein with relatively clean ingredients. Many cans have pull-tops, which make them great for travel.

Among my favorite finds that provide protein and/or fat:

- canned chicken
- canned ground beef
- canned pulled pork
- canned salmon
- canned shrimp
- canned tuna
- frozen precooked chicken (some brands contain less-than-ideal ingredients, but this is a reasonable option when you're in a hurry)
- individual pouches of pepperoni
- single-serving frozen chicken, shrimp, and fish (which require cooking)

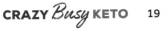

Also, as you travel, you can often find free condiments to help you create on-the-go meals. Packets of mayonnaise, mustard, and vinegar can be used to make an impromptu egg salad and are often available from delis, grocery store food bars, convenience stores that sell hot dogs or sandwiches, and even fast-food restaurants. I've also found packets of cream cheese and peanut butter at stores that sell bagels and at hotel breakfast bars. The cream cheese provides an excellent boost in fat when added to eggs. I've even used chopped nuts and cream cheese with a few berries to make a treat at breakfast when few keto-friendly options were available. Packets of peanut butter can be mixed with cream cheese and/or butter to make a quick fat bomb.

Keep your eyes open as you travel. You may find more options than you ever thought possible!

# CRAZY BUSY RESTAURANT GUIDE

Dining out can be daunting if you're used to eating at home. Whether you're turning to a restaurant for convenience or for a well-deserved break from the kitchen, knowing what to order can help.

Let's be honest: as much as I prefer to cook homemade meals for my family, there are times when doing so simply isn't possible. When we do find ourselves ordering out, we are generally facing one of three situations:

1. We are traveling.

2. We are socializing.

3. Plans B, C, D, and E fell through, and there were simply no other options (although, admittedly, a restaurant can be a decent Plan B option).

Regardless, when you are following a keto diet, some restaurant meals are better than others.

## TAKEOUT MEALS

If you find yourself needing to place a keto-friendly order for a quick meal on the run, here are a few ideas:

- **Bunless burgers**—Fast, inexpensive, and easy to find! I typically add bacon and cheese. Avoid chili because it may contain food starches and could cause intestinal distress. Top your burger with mayo, tomato, pickles, and/or mustard; avoid ketchup and "special sauces" because of the added sugar. Order your burger without the bun to avoid temptation and so that the cheese doesn't stick to the bun. Restaurants are more likely to include utensils with your to-go order if the burger is not lettuce wrapped. I usually ask for my burger in a tray so that it's easier to eat.

- **Fajitas**—Order for two, with extra guacamole and sour cream—hold the rice, beans, and tortillas. That's all you need to know! My family orders this meal at least once a month, most frequently asking for a mix of chicken, beef, Mexican chorizo (spicy sausage), and carnitas (pork). Fajitas come with sautéed vegetables, most often onions and bell peppers. I recommend avoiding queso, as it often contains added flour and thickeners. Shredded cheese is usually a better option. With added guacamole, sour cream, and cheese, this is a complete meal.

  Also, we intentionally order more fajitas than we expect to eat. The leftovers are perfect for lunches the following day. Even when there are few leftovers, you can add the remaining meat and veggies to a 2-Minute Microwave Omelet (page 40) for a very good morning!

- **Wings**—As long as they are unbreaded and not bathed in a sweet sauce, chicken wings are a great takeout meal. You can season them yourself at home. (See pages 70 to 73 for three of my favorite options.)

- **BBQ or smoked meats**—We frequently order these types of meats by the pound, especially when traveling. Pulled pork, brisket, or smoked chicken becomes a complete meal when paired with a salad or a simple low-carb veggie, or simply dipped in a fatty sauce! You can also toss the leftovers into an omelet.

  If I find myself with more meat than we will reasonably eat in a week, I freeze the excess in single-serving portions. They can be eaten as meals or added to soups or stews for flavor or protein.

## SIT-DOWN MEALS

When we're not eating on the run, but rather enjoying a full meal at a sit-down restaurant for relaxation or socializing, we choose dishes that may take a bit more time to prepare. Among our standbys:

- **Grilled meat with a side salad and extra dressing**—Nearly always an option regardless of the type of restaurant.

- **Steak with loaded broccoli**—Just ask for the sour cream, bacon, cheese, and butter that normally would be added to a baked potato to be added to steamed broccoli instead. You're welcome!

- **Seafood with butter and a simple low-carb side, such as asparagus, broccoli, or spinach**—Make sure that the seafood is not coated in flour or cornmeal, and ask for extra butter.

- **Mexican dishes**—In addition to the fajitas I mentioned above, dishes featuring carnitas, grilled chicken or beef, and veggies are usually great options. We like to add chorizo for additional flavor and fat. Refuse the chips and tortillas.

Italian restaurants don't have to be off-limits, either. Many times the meats and sauces usually served over pasta can be served over sautéed spinach instead. Seafood, steaks, and grilled meats are common at many Italian restaurants and are very satisfying when paired with a nice salad. A caprese salad with an antipasto platter (check the appetizer menu) is a perfect meal for me!

While there are few types of restaurants that I avoid completely, the exception is Asian restaurants, which generally offer few good keto options. Occasionally, you can find reasonable seafood or meat choices, but many lack the fat that you would want for satiety. The sauces are also likely to be sweetened with sugar, and there are generally few low-carb sides offered.

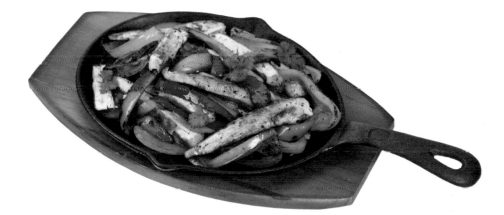

## KETO SALADS

Don't fall into the diet mentality of ordering a salad, as a salad may not be the best choice for a ketogenic meal. The problem is that salads often contain little protein and few fats, but lots of carbs. If you find yourself perusing the salads, build a better salad with

- **Sources of protein:** bacon, other meats, eggs, nuts, cheese

- **Sources of fat:** avocado, fatty dressing, bacon, cheese

When choosing a salad dressing, keep in mind that options such as ranch and blue cheese are often mayonnaise based, low in sugar, and high in fat. Avoid sweet dressings such as French, Thousand Island, and honey mustard. Citrusy vinaigrettes are often loaded with sugar or honey. Be sure to ask the server about the ingredients. If there are no acceptable premade dressings, most restaurants offer the simple option of olive oil and vinegar that you can drizzle over your salad at the table.

Limit carbs by being careful with common salad veggies, such as broccoli, carrots, cucumbers, onions, and tomatoes. Avoid beans, corn, croutons, sweetened nuts, and wheat-based toppings such as French-fried onions. Ignore any bread, rolls, or crackers served with the salad. You might ask the server to remove the bread from the table or place it on a dirty plate to help you avoid temptation. You can also offer it to someone else at the table with a casual "I don't care for this. Would you like it?" If the bread is talking to you, get rid of it fast to shut it up!

# NAVIGATING THE RECIPES

At the tops of the recipes, I've included a few icons to help you find what you need:

No kitchen needed

Microwaveable

Can be prepped ahead

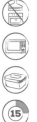 Can be prepped in under 15 minutes

Can be prepped in under 30 minutes

Dairy-free*

Nut-free*

*If preceded by the word *option,* the recipe can be made dairy/nut-free with modifications.

# FINALLY

Even though I keep thinking that life will come at me in a slower pace when the next project is finished or when school lets out for summer or when school begins again, those leisurely times never seem to materialize. Whether it's work, school, family, or friends, life can come at us fast.

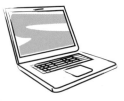

Many of us don't have the luxury of waiting until we have time to focus on getting healthy. We have to find ways to get or stay healthy while making time for the crazy busy, wonderful stuff that most of us call life!

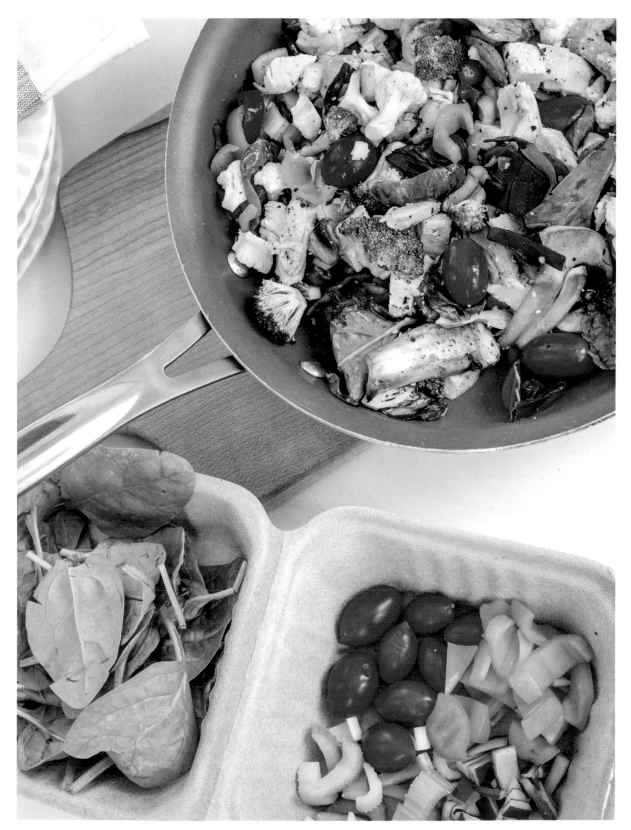

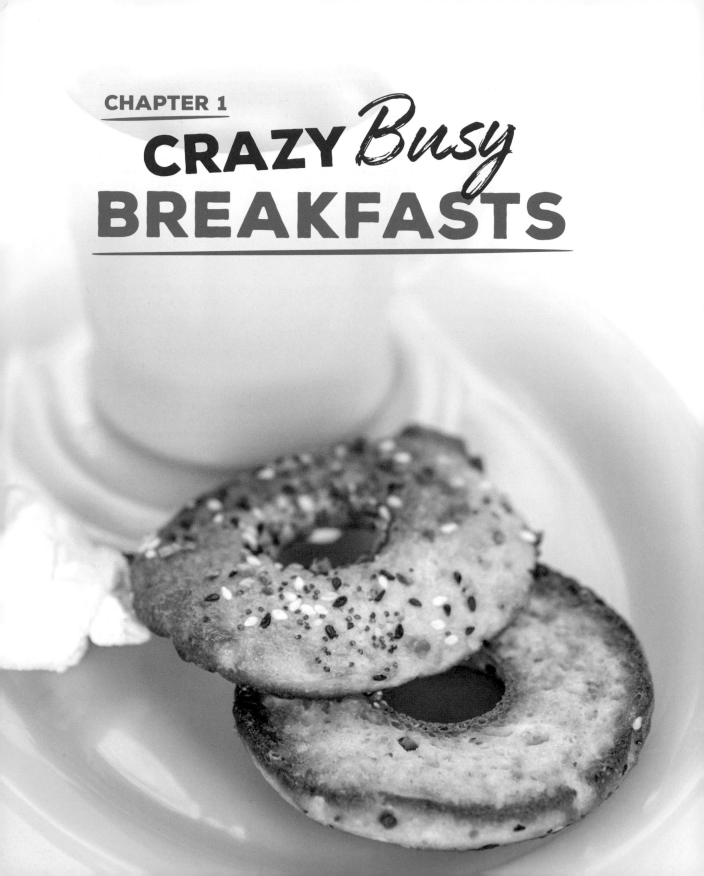

# CHAPTER 1
## CRAZY *Busy*
## BREAKFASTS

Arguably, breakfast can be the single most challenging meal of the day. Who has the time to sit down to eat a morning meal even if there was time to prepare one? With the occasional exception on weekends, most of my breakfasts are eaten standing, walking, driving, or in bites between computer clicks at my desk. And I suspect I'm not alone in those habits.

For this reason, I begin this chapter with six super fast meals that aren't really recipes as much as they are ideas for quick meals that have a great balance of fat and protein and very low carbs. These don't necessarily have to be prepped ahead of time, although some of them can be. Most can be grabbed on the way out of the house, stored in an office fridge, or easily eaten during a commute. Because no cooking is required, they may be great options for children, too.

The recipes that I've included in this chapter are either quick and easy or prepped ahead of time so that they're ready when you need to eat. Before you scoff at the idea of prepping ahead, here's an example of how I make meal prep as painless as possible. Sunday is the one night of the week when we are nearly always home. While I'm already in the kitchen making dinner, I toss together one of those very quick breakfast recipes that need to be baked. Frittatas, muffins, or bagels are perfect examples. The dish bakes while we eat dinner. Once it's ready, I remove it from the oven. By the time I'm nearly finished cleaning the kitchen, the frittata, muffins, or bagels have cooled and are ready to be stored in the fridge. To make mornings go even more smoothly, I sometimes portion the frittata or slice the bagels in half. The next morning, my future self will thank me!

Some people make breakfast even easier to manage by skipping it altogether. It doesn't get much faster than grabbing a cup of coffee or a glass of ice water (which I often crave in the morning) and heading out the door. When I do this, I wait until I'm hungry to eat. Some days it's midmorning, and other days it's midday or even dinnertime. The old notion of eating breakfast to jump-start our metabolism simply isn't accurate; our bodies can thrive while having ample time to use our on-board reserves. However, if you wake up hungry, there are plenty of quick and easy options to have you fueled and ready for the day.

Keep in mind that breakfast food can be anything. My daughter nearly always eats leftovers. She doesn't care whether it's Italian, Mexican, or deli meat with cheese and mayo. Break free from those old notions that cereals and grains are good and that breakfast is reserved for eggs and bacon, although I'll admit that a simple egg scrambled in butter and paired with a few strips of bacon is about as perfect a meal as you'll ever eat.

As you read through this chapter, keep an eye out for the Crazy Busy Travel Tips for breakfasts that can be made using little more than a microwave. Also, notice that you can mix and match the breakfast meal ideas according to what you like or have access to. As discussed on pages 17 to 19, traveling on keto is often easier than you might think, especially if you can stop at a convenience store or grocery store along the way.

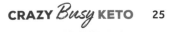

# MEAL *Ideas*

Though not technically recipes, here are a few very quick and super tasty breakfast options that my family eats from time to time. If you refer to the lists on pages 12 to 16, you'll see the ingredients that I nearly always have on hand. We pull a variety of items from that list but often fall back on precooked bacon when there's little else. If our supply falls below one full warehouse club–sized package, then we declare an emergency! Not only are these quick meals for grabbing at home, but they are perfect for traveling or camping as well.

## BACON AND GUACAMOLE

While ingredients vary by brand, there are a few brands of single-serving guacamole cups that have excellent ingredients and are truly low-carb. These won't turn brown and are perfect portions for meals. When paired with precooked bacon, guacamole makes truly a fast and easy meal, and the macros are excellent, with the guacamole cups offering roughly 11 grams of fat and 4 total carbs and 4 slices of precooked bacon providing about 5 grams of protein and 6 grams of fat! Don't be afraid to eat extra bacon to get sufficient protein Keep in mind that the nutritional values of products will vary, so be sure to check the labels for the brands you use.

## HARD-BOILED EGGS, CREAM CHEESE, AND BACON PIECES

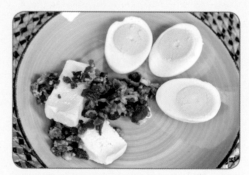

Hard-boiled eggs are a great breakfast option. You can either boil up a batch in advance or buy them already boiled and peeled in a package. Some convenience stores even sell them in small packs of two. Pairing the eggs with cream cheese and bacon pieces adds just enough fat and flavor to make the eggs more satiating. Eggs provide great nutrition with 6 grams of protein, 5 grams of fat, and 0.6 gram of carbs in each egg. One tablespoon of bacon pieces, which come in travel packs, adds 3 grams of protein and 1.5 grams of fat, while 1 tablespoon of cream cheese has 1 gram of protein, 5 grams of fat, and no carbs.

## PRECOOKED SAUSAGE AND CHEESE

Pork breakfast sausage is available in links as well as patties. You can also buy sausage made from grass-fed beef that has pretty good ingredients. I prefer to cook up a batch of sausage patties on the weekend or when I'm cooking double (see page 7), but precooked sausages will do during an exceptionally busy time or when I'm traveling. The nutritional information will vary widely among brands; I tend to use those with no sugar or fillers, which are often labeled "natural." A cooked sausage patty will yield roughly 5 grams of protein and 8 grams of fat. An ounce of cheese will add fat and protein, with the exact amount depending on the type of cheese you choose. Most cheddar cheeses have about 5 grams of protein, 7 grams of fat, and less than 1 gram of carbs per ounce.

## CHEESE CRISPS, BACON, GRAPE TOMATOES, AND RANCH

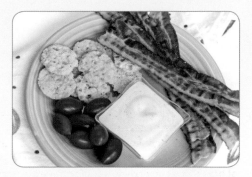

Those addictive little cheese crackers, aka "crisps," often can be found in single-serving packages. When paired with bacon, grape tomatoes, and ranch dressing, it feels more like a real meal. And if you haven't tried bacon dipped in ranch dressing, then you are welcome! I tend to count grape tomatoes as 1 gram of carbs each, especially if they are large. The crisps I use provide 13 grams of protein and 11 grams of fat per 1-ounce serving, and 4 slices of precooked bacon add 5 grams of protein and 6 grams of fat. My homemade ranch dressing has more protein and fat than the store-bought travel cups of ranch dressing, which have 13 grams of fat, a trace amount of protein, and 2 grams of carbs per 1-ounce serving.

## EVERYTHING BAGEL BREAKFAST SANDWICH

Let's be honest: a breakfast sandwich equals a little freedom when on the run. No knife and fork, just clean hands and a good, hot meal! My low-carb keto Everything Bagels (page 36) make breakfast sandwiches a real thing again. These bagels are as sturdy as they are tasty. Use your imagination to find your favorite sandwich combos. I often pair scrambled eggs with bacon, fried eggs with breakfast sausage, or sausage with the first scrap of cheese I grab from the fridge. Precooked bacon or sausage is ideal for making a bagel breakfast sandwich on the fly since there is nothing to cook. Also, don't forget to step out of the box and try fillings such as chicken salad or egg salad, or opt for the traditional ham and cheese.

Although I've placed them in the breakfast chapter, my Everything Bagels can be tossed in a lunch box or used as a bun for a burger at dinner, too.

## WAFFLE BREAKFAST SANDWICH

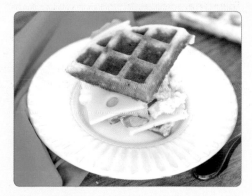

My homemade waffles are also sturdy enough to serve as a great "bun" for a sandwich on a busy morning. You can modify the waffle recipe to make your breakfast sandwich with a sweet or savory waffle "bun" (see Note, page 43). While you can use any sandwich fillings you want, I like a fried or scrambled egg, cheese (to hold it together), and some bacon, ham, or breakfast sausage patties (all precooked, of course!). A schmear of cream cheese is fantastic, too.

To make one sandwich, take ½ Crazy Busy Waffle (page 42) and toast it in a toaster or skillet. Separate the warmed half waffle into two quarters and use them as the top and bottom "bun" for your sandwich.

*Crazy Busy Kitchen Tip:* *If you don't have a good way to warm the half waffle or enough time to warm it, it is still a great option for making a breakfast sandwich, even when taken straight from the fridge.*

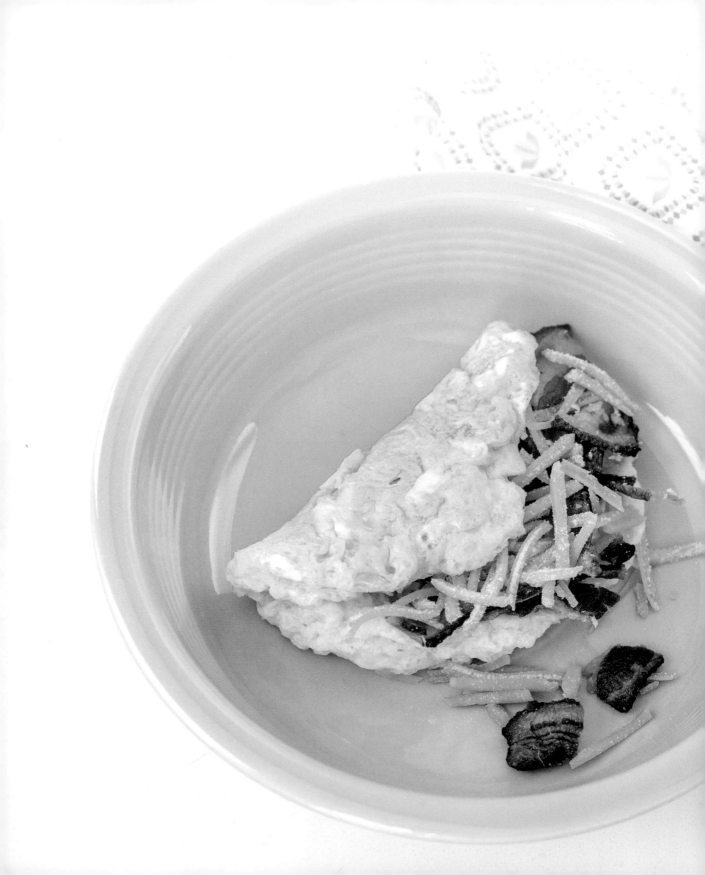

# Recipes

# GOOD MORNING GRANOLA

OPTION

**MAKES** 10 servings (½ cup per serving)
**PREP TIME:** 18 minutes, plus 1½ hours to cool  |  **COOK TIME:** 45 minutes

*We love this stuff! Even my husband, who doesn't love coconut flakes and despises pork rinds, enjoys this granola. The pork rinds are what keep it low-carb while adding a respectable amount of fat and protein. And while it isn't fast to make because of the baking time, it is fast to toss together, and you can do other things while it bakes on low heat. Just be sure to set a timer so you don't forget to give it a stir every 15 to 20 minutes. I've also left it in the oven with the door ajar overnight, which makes it even crispier and means that I wake to fresh, warm granola. See my tip below for making a low-carb milk substitute that renders this a perfect breakfast. You can also add a tablespoon or two of hemp hearts to give the granola a nice texture as well as additional protein and omega-3 fats. While I tend to store this cereal in the fridge since it has no preservatives, it travels well and doesn't have to be refrigerated during travel.*

**2 cups broken pork rind pieces (about 1 ounce)**

**1 cup unsweetened coconut flakes**

**¾ cup raw almonds**

**½ cup raw pecan pieces**

**½ cup chopped raw walnuts**

**¼ cup raw pumpkin seeds**

**3 tablespoons granulated sweetener**

**2 tablespoons ground cinnamon**

**½ teaspoon salt**

**1 large egg white, room temperature**

**⅓ cup unsalted butter, melted but not hot (use coconut oil for dairy-free)**

**2 teaspoons vanilla extract**

**5 drops liquid sweetener**

1. Preheat the oven to 250°F. Line a rimmed baking sheet with parchment paper or aluminum foil, then lightly grease the paper or foil and set aside.

2. In a large bowl, toss the pork rind pieces with the coconut flakes, almonds, pecans, walnuts, and pumpkin seeds.

3. In a small bowl, mix together the granulated sweetener, cinnamon, and salt.

4. In another small bowl, whip the egg white until frothy. Add the melted butter, vanilla extract, and liquid sweetener. Pour the egg white mixture over the pork rind mixture, tossing to coat evenly. Be sure that each piece is lightly coated. Next, sprinkle the cinnamon mixture over the pork rind mixture and toss to distribute.

5. Spread the granola in a single layer on the prepared baking sheet. Bake for 45 to 50 minutes, stirring every 15 to 20 minutes, until lightly browned. Turn off the oven and let the granola cool in the oven with the door ajar for at least 1½ hours. For crunchier granola, let it sit longer. Store in an airtight container in the refrigerator for up to 2 weeks.

*Cook's Notes:* Using raw nuts and seeds is best, as they will roast while the granola is baking. If you begin with roasted nuts, they may become overbaked.

Make sure that the egg white is at room temperature before adding the melted butter, or the cold egg white will cause the butter to solidify. Also, egg whites whip better at room temperature.

For morning cereal without the sugars in dairy milk, mix 2 tablespoons of heavy cream with ¼ cup of unsweetened almond milk and pour over a ½-cup serving of granola. This blend of cream and almond milk more closely resembles full-fat dairy milk than any other substitute I've tried.

Calories: 298 | Fat: 32g | Protein: 12g | Carbs: 5.9g | Fiber: 3.8g | Erythritol: 6g

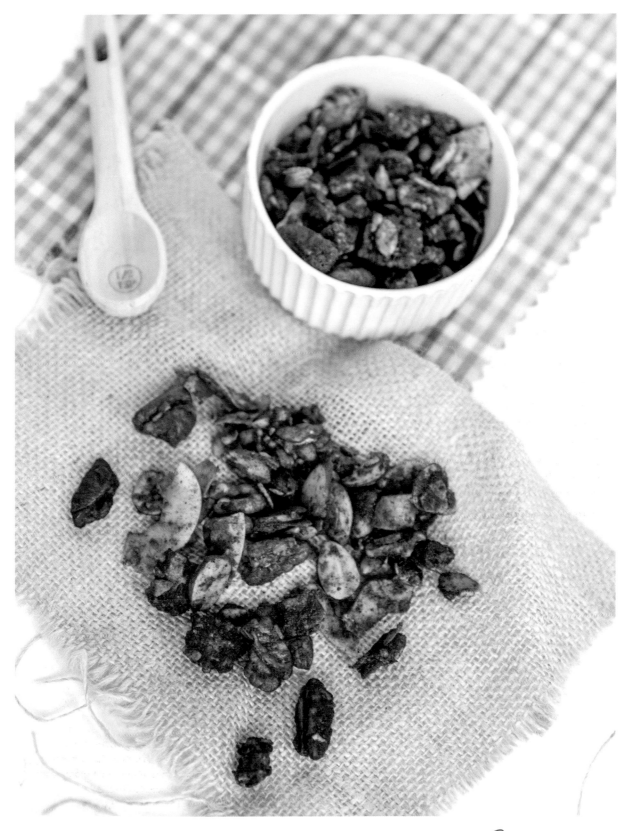

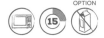

# LEMON MINUTE MUFFINS

OPTION

**MAKES** 2 muffins (1 per serving)
**PREP TIME:** 4 minutes, plus 5 minutes to cool | **COOK TIME:** 1 minute

*If morning sunshine is yellow, then these muffins are morning sunshine! I love the taste of lemon, and these muffins are like a dose of sunshine served up in moist muffin form. Yes, they are moist. In fact, I had to tweak the recipe a few times to make them less moist. The muffins are cooked in a microwave to make it quick, but a little prep work can make them even easier to enjoy on a hectic morning. First, you can make them ahead of time. I've cooked them in ramekins, covered them with a lid or plastic wrap, and eaten them the next day, either cold or warmed in the microwave on reduced power for about 20 seconds. You can also save time by mixing the dry ingredients ahead of time. The dry mix can be stored in a jar or plastic bag in the fridge for up to 4 weeks or the freezer for up to 3 months. Simply add the egg, lemon juice, and melted butter and prepare according to the instructions below. This is an especially simple recipe for children to prepare, but be sure to warn them to use an oven mitt or cloth to remove the muffins from the microwave; the containers will be hot. Also, you can use ramekins, small bowls, or even coffee mugs to make these muffins.*

**3 tablespoons blanched almond flour**

**2 tablespoons granulated sweetener**

**1 tablespoon coconut flour**

**½ teaspoon baking powder**

**1 large egg, beaten**

**2 tablespoons lemon juice**

**1 tablespoon unsalted butter, melted (use coconut oil for dairy-free)**

1. Grease two microwave-safe 8-ounce ramekins or coffee mugs.

2. In a small mixing bowl, whisk together the dry ingredients. Add the egg, lemon juice, and melted butter and whisk until smooth. Divide the batter between the ramekins.

3. Microwave both ramekins together on high for 1 minute. If the muffins are not set, microwave in additional 20-second bursts until just firm and set. Use an oven mitt or towel to remove them from the microwave and let cool for at least 5 minutes. The muffins will firm up and dry out as they cool. You can eat your muffin directly from the ramekin or mug with a spoon or loosen the edges with a knife and invert it onto a small plate. Store leftovers in the refrigerator for up to 1 week.

*Crazy Busy Kitchen Tip:* Grease the ramekins and melt the butter at the same time by placing ½ tablespoon of butter in each ramekin and microwaving on reduced power for 10 to 15 seconds, or until the butter is melted. Be careful, or the butter may pop and make a mess in the microwave if heated too long. Swirl the melted butter around the ramekins to coat the sides and bottoms, then pour the excess into the mixing bowl with the dry ingredients and continue making the batter.

*Crazy Busy Travel Tip:* Take the dry ingredients with you. All you need is an egg, lemon juice, and butter. A six-pack of eggs fits easily in a hotel mini fridge and often can be purchased at convenience stores, which also carry butter. I've also shamelessly asked for butter and extra lemon wedges at restaurants. It takes only three or four wedges to yield enough juice for this recipe. You can mix the batter in a cup and use the coffee mugs provided in the room to microwave the muffins. If there is no microwave in the room, many hotels have microwaves in the breakfast or common area.

**Calories:** 222 | **Fat:** 16.1g | **Protein:** 5.6g | **Carbs:** 6.9g | **Fiber:** 4.2g | **Erythritol:** 8g

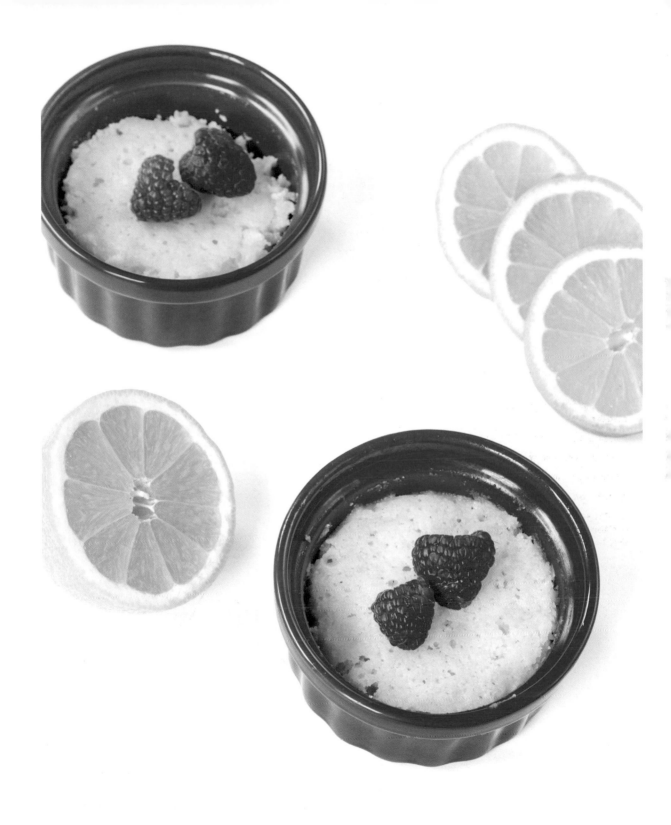

# LOCO MOCHA MUFFINS

**MAKES** 12 muffins (1 per serving)
**PREP TIME:** 8 minutes, plus 5 minutes to cool | **COOK TIME:** 20 minutes

*In this case, loco stands for "low-carb"! You'd be crazy not to make these muffins. They are easily prepped ahead and make a quick breakfast on the go. I like them warmed with a little softened butter, cream cheese, or bacon for added protein. The hint of coffee flavor makes the chocolate perfectly acceptable for mornings. If you prefer chocolate without the mocha flavor, you can omit the coffee powder. You can also get a double hit of chocolate by adding a few low-carb chocolate chips.*

1⅔ cups blanched almond flour

½ cup unsweetened cocoa powder

2 teaspoons instant coffee powder or espresso powder

1 teaspoon baking powder

½ teaspoon salt

½ cup (1 stick) unsalted butter, softened

2 ounces cream cheese (¼ cup), softened

¾ cup granulated sweetener

3 large eggs

⅓ cup refined coconut oil (see note), melted but not hot

¼ cup heavy cream

2 teaspoons vanilla extract

8 drops liquid sweetener

1. Preheat the oven to 350°F. Line a standard-size 12-well muffin pan with parchment paper liners.

2. In a medium bowl, whisk together the almond flour, cocoa powder, coffee powder, baking powder, and salt, making sure the ingredients are well mixed.

3. In a large mixing bowl, use a hand mixer to cream the butter, cream cheese, and granulated sweetener. Beat in the eggs, melted coconut oil, heavy cream, vanilla extract, and liquid sweetener. Add the dry ingredients to the wet ingredients and mix well by hand.

4. Divide the batter evenly among the wells of the muffin pan, filling each about two-thirds full. Bake for 20 to 22 minutes, or until a toothpick inserted in the center of a muffin comes out clean. Do not overbake or the muffins will be dry and crumbly.

5. Let the muffins cool in the pan for 5 to 10 minutes before serving. Store leftovers in the refrigerator for up to 1 week or in the freezer for up to 3 months—they are excellent frozen.

*Cook's Note:* Because my husband despises the flavor of coconut, I use refined coconut oil, which has a milder taste, unless I'm making a coconut-flavored dessert.

*Crazy Busy Kitchen Tip:* Like other baked goods in this book, the dry ingredients can be combined in advance and refrigerated until you are ready to mix them with the wet ingredients.

*Crazy Busy Travel Tip:* Make these muffins made ahead and freeze them individually. When you're ready to hit the road, grab one out of the freezer. It will thaw as you travel and makes a perfect traveling companion!

Calories: 178 | Fat: 18.8g | Protein: 2.2g | Carbs: 3.3g | Fiber: 1.6g | Erythritol: 8g

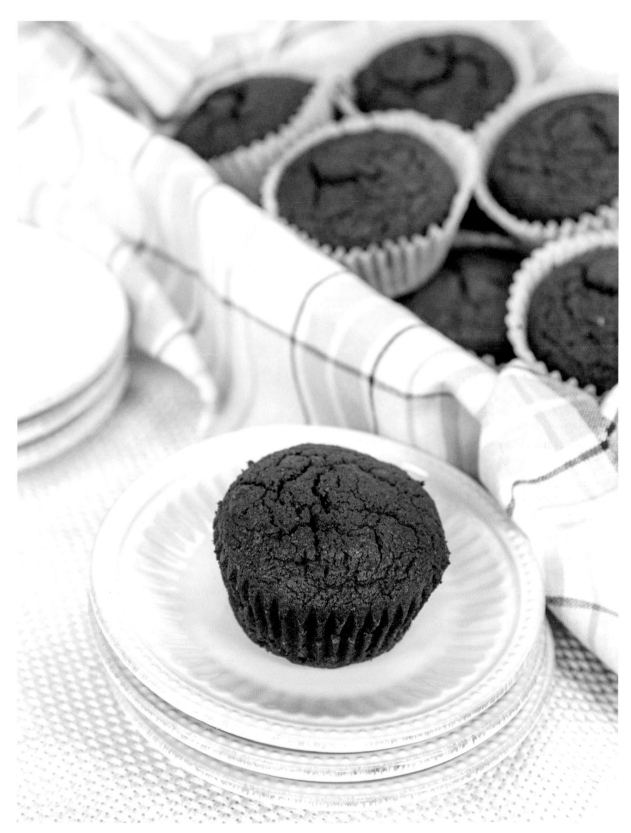

# EVERYTHING BAGELS

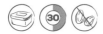

**MAKES** 6 bagels (1 per serving)
**PREP TIME:** 8 minutes, plus 15 minutes to cool | **COOK TIME:** 15 minutes

*These are my favorite bagels. Even though they aren't as chewy as traditional New York bagels, adding the psyllium fiber gives them that distinctive chew that is often missing from low-carb baked goods. These make a great breakfast smeared with cream cheese or butter or sliced and used for a breakfast sandwich (see page 27). I love using the Everything but the Bagel seasoning available from Trader Joe's, but you can easily make your own.*

**2 tablespoons everything bagel seasoning, divided**

**3 ounces mozzarella cheese, shredded (about ¾ cup), room temperature**

**2 ounces shredded Parmesan cheese, room temperature**

**2 ounces cream cheese (¼ cup), softened**

**2 large egg whites**

**½ cup unflavored whey protein isolate**

**1½ tablespoons psyllium fiber**

**1 teaspoon baking powder**

**¼ teaspoon garlic powder**

**¼ teaspoon onion powder**

**½ teaspoon salt (omit if the cheeses are salty)**

**⅓ cup very hot water**

**3 tablespoons melted ghee or unsalted butter**

**SPECIAL EQUIPMENT:**

**6-well doughnut pan**

1. Preheat the oven to 350°F. Grease a 6-well doughnut pan and sprinkle 1 tablespoon of the everything bagel seasoning evenly into the wells.

2. Mix together the cheeses and egg whites in a mixing bowl and set aside. In a separate bowl, stir together the whey protein isolate, psyllium fiber, baking powder, garlic powder, onion powder, and salt, if using. While stirring to prevent the psyllium from clumping, add the hot water to the dry ingredients. When the water is absorbed, add the cheese mixture and melted ghee to the psyllium mixture and stir well. The batter will be very thick, but much thinner than a traditional bagel dough.

3. Distribute the batter evenly among the prepared wells of the doughnut pan, filling each nearly to the top. Evenly sprinkle the remaining 1 tablespoon of everything bagel seasoning over the tops.

4. Bake for 15 to 17 minutes, or until the bagels are browned and firm to the touch. Let cool for 15 to 20 minutes before removing from the pan and placing on a cooling rack to finish cooling. When completely cool, use a serrated knife to slice the bagels. They toast best when you use the oven broiler or the broil setting in a toaster oven.

5. Store leftovers in the refrigerator for up to 6 days, or wrap sliced bagels individually in freezer paper, place in a plastic freezer bag, and freeze for up to 3 months. To use, remove from the freezer, separate the slices, and toast using the broiler setting.

*Crazy Busy Kitchen Tip:* These bagels truly take less than 30 minutes to toss together once you're familiar with the recipe. You can also store the dry ingredients in an airtight container in the refrigerator for up to a week. Having the dry mix available means that you can throw them together and bake the bagels while you're enjoying dinner or washing dishes.

*Crazy Busy Travel Tip:* Take one of these bagels with you for your drive-through bunless burger order. It makes eating a burger in the car much easier than using a knife and fork or a messy, drippy lettuce wrap. You can also let the bagels thaw at room temperature for travel.

**Calories:** 265 | **Fat:** 13.6g | **Protein:** 15.9g | **Carbs:** 3.6g | **Fiber:** 2.4g

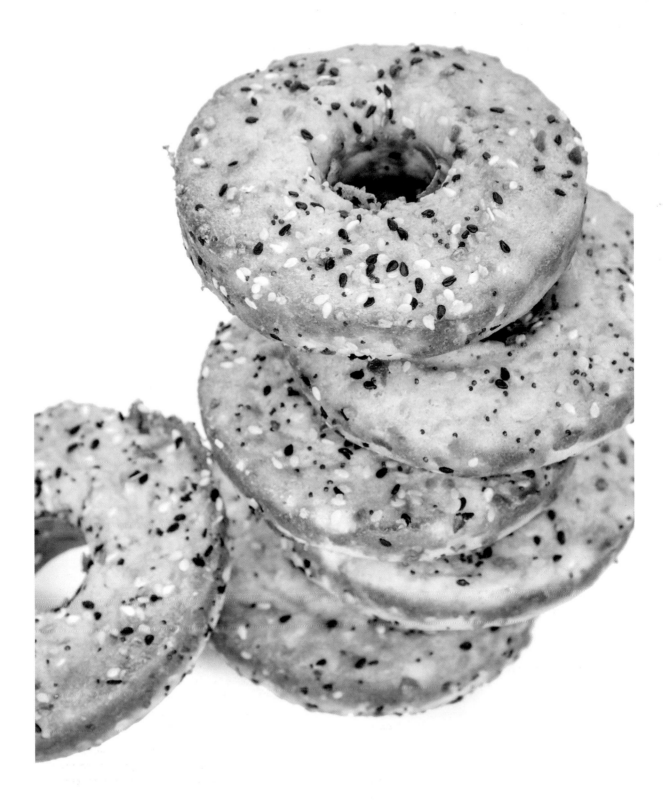

# SALAD BAR CRUSTLESS QUICHE

**MAKES** 6 servings
**PREP TIME:** 6 minutes, plus 10 minutes to set | **COOK TIME:** 30 minutes

*Crazy Busy Keto works because of simple shortcuts, such as using items you "find" in the fridge, stocking your kitchen with items that are shelf-stable or freezer-friendly, and buying prepared or precooked items that you can grab quickly. For this recipe, I used frozen asparagus that was thawed, patted dry, and chopped, but you could just as easily use chopped canned asparagus or fresh asparagus from the salad bar. I also used ham that was already cubed (often shelved with the breakfast meats in the refrigerated section of the grocery store), so I didn't have to chop it. Using dried minced onion, which has an excellent shelf life, saves you the time of chopping an onion, but you can use fresh onion if you prefer. Green onion is especially tasty in this quiche. As discussed on page 8, the salad bar is a great place to grab small amounts of ingredients that are already cleaned and prepped. Feel free to be creative and create your own crustless quiche using ingredients such as bell peppers, broccoli, celery, grape tomatoes, mushrooms, onion, or spinach; just be sure to keep the amount of cheese, eggs, and cream the same.*

**10 to 12 asparagus spears, trimmed and chopped**

**1 cup cubed cooked ham**

**4 ounces cheddar cheese, shredded (about 1 cup)**

**1 tablespoon dried minced onion**

**5 large eggs**

**1 cup heavy cream**

**½ teaspoon salt**

1. Preheat the oven to 350°F. Grease a 9-inch glass pie pan with butter.

2. Evenly distribute the asparagus, ham, cheese, and dried minced onion in the prepared pie pan and set aside.

3. In a large bowl, whisk together the eggs, cream, and salt until frothy. Pour the whisked egg mixture over the ingredients in the pie pan.

4. Bake for 30 to 35 minutes, or until the center of the quiche is just set and lightly browned. Remove from the oven and let set for 10 to 15 minutes before serving.

5. If storing for later use, let cool to room temperature, slice into 6 equal portions, and store in an airtight container in the refrigerator until ready to eat. Warm it on reduced power in the microwave, if desired, or eat it chilled. Store leftovers in the refrigerator for up to 1 week.

Calories: 283 | Fat: 19.9g | Protein: 20.3g | Carbs: 5.8g | Fiber: 0.9g

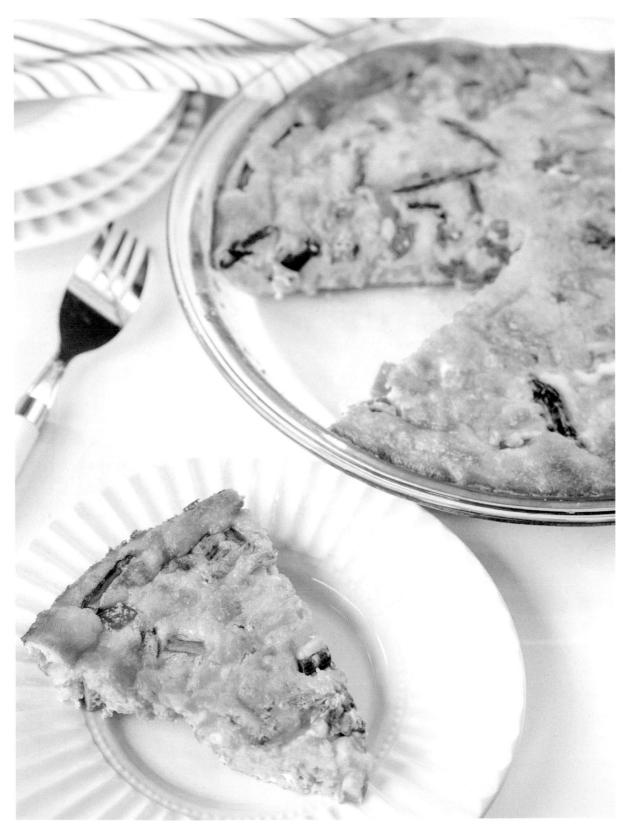

# 2-MINUTE MICROWAVE OMELET

**MAKES** 1 serving | **PREP TIME:** 4 minutes (not including time to cook bacon if not purchased precooked) | **COOK TIME:** 2 minutes

*I call this a "found" omelet because you make it from anything you can find! I love making these and often find myself preparing one for a quick and nutritious breakfast, lunch, or even dinner. You can do cooked chicken, spinach, and feta; a classic (and easy) ham and cheese; or simply cheese and precooked bacon. I also enjoy using leftovers for this recipe. Carnitas with a few peppers and onions are perfect, as is leftover steak, taco meat, fajitas, or precooked sausage. You can add nearly any cheese imaginable. I've used Swiss, Havarti, Monterey Jack, jalapeño Jack, Gouda, cheddar, and even Parmesan. Veggies are always optional, but I generally use leftover veggies that are already cooked, such as broccoli, mushrooms, onions, peppers, or zucchini. Raw veggies such as spinach or tomatoes are good as well. Also, I tend to use only one egg so that the egg layer isn't too thick. You can use two if you prefer, but the omelet part will be thicker and may be harder to fold. (In that case, simply eat it straight from the bowl!) The only limit is your imagination.*

**1 tablespoon salted butter or refined coconut oil**

**1 large egg**

**1 ounce cheddar cheese, shredded or cubed (omit for dairy-free)**

**1 ounce bacon (about 1 strip), cooked and chopped**

**Dash of salt**

**Dash of ground black pepper**

1. Grease a standard-size microwave-safe cereal or soup bowl with the butter and set aside. In a glass or a small bowl, beat the egg with a fork until well blended. Pour the egg into the buttered bowl.

2. Microwave for up to 1 minute, or until set in the center. Carefully remove the bowl from the microwave; it will be hot.

3. Add the cheese and bacon (or your preferred fillings). Microwave for an additional 15 to 20 seconds, or until the fillings are heated through. Remove from the microwave, fold one half over the over like a traditional omelet, sprinkle with the salt and pepper, and serve immediately. These omelets can also be made ahead of time and warmed on reduced power.

*Crazy Busy Kitchen Tip:* Microwave the omelet in a paper bowl. You can eat it straight out of the bowl and then dispose of the bowl, leaving you with minimal cleanup.

*Crazy Busy Travel Tip:* You can easily make these omelets on the road as long as you have access to a microwave. When traveling, I like to buy string cheese or other cheese sticks (such as cheddar, Gouda, or Monterey Jack) to use in this recipe. Cheese sticks don't contain the food starches used in preshredded cheese. Because they are individually packaged, I can eat them as a snack, as part of my traveling lunch, or to create a breakfast like this one! See pages 17 to 19 for more travel ideas.

Calories: 437 | Fat: 37.3g | Protein: 23.9g | Carbs: 0.8g | Fiber: 0g

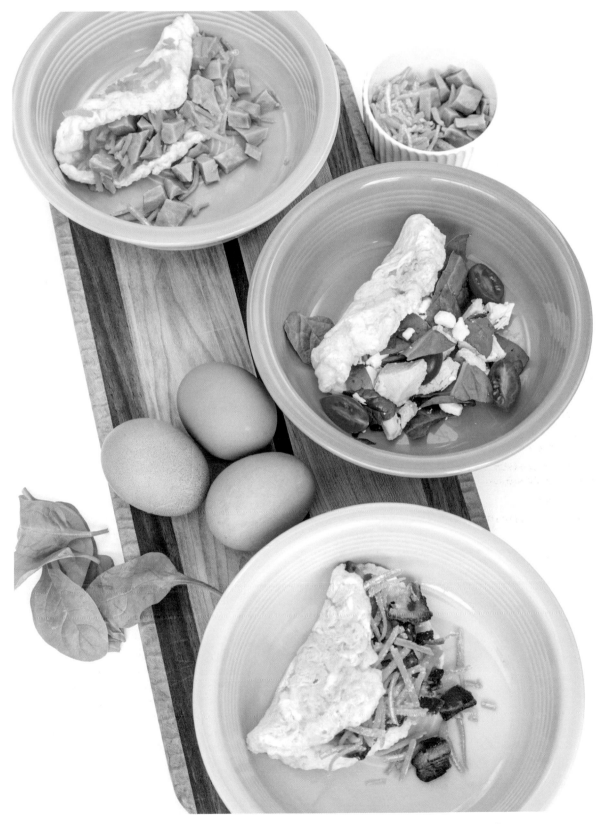

# CRAZY BUSY WAFFLES

**MAKES** 4 waffles (½ per serving)
**PREP TIME:** 4 minutes  |  **COOK TIME:** 12 minutes

*Did you read that right? A serving is half of a waffle? These waffles are super filling, and while you might want to eat an entire waffle, I find that half really is enough. Plus, it's the perfect size for making a breakfast sandwich! Full disclaimer: these waffles are not crisp, even when toasted. Still, what makes them ideal is that they are sturdy and flavorful and easily made ahead of time for a breakfast that defies the traditional notion of "diet." If you choose to use coconut flour instead of pork rind dust, the waffles will be even softer. Also, you want to use a low setting on the waffle maker. Like other low-carb foods, these waffles are softer when first made and firm up quickly. In fact, I have turned off my waffle maker and waited 30 seconds before using a pair of rubber-tipped tongs to remove the waffle, which gives it time to become a bit sturdier.*

**2 ounces cream cheese (¼ cup)**

**¼ cup granulated sweetener (see Note)**

**⅓ cup pork rind dust, or 2 tablespoons coconut flour**

**½ cup blanched almond flour**

**1 teaspoon baking powder**

**1 teaspoon vanilla extract**

**4 large eggs**

**Simple Pancake Syrup, for serving (optional; see recipe below)**

1.  Preheat a waffle maker to low heat per the manufacturer's instructions.

2.  Soften the cream cheese in a microwave-safe mixing bowl in the microwave. Add the remaining ingredients and use a rubber spatula or whisk to mix the ingredients thoroughly. When the waffle maker is ready, pour in ½ cup of the batter, close the lid, and cook until the waffle is golden brown. Carefully remove the waffle using rubber-tipped tongs or a spatula. It may be fragile until cool. Repeat with the remaining batter.

3.  Serve immediately with the pancake syrup, if desired, or let cool on a cooling rack if you intend to store the waffles for later use. Store the waffles in the refrigerator for up to 6 days or in the freezer for up to 2 months.

# SIMPLE PANCAKE SYRUP

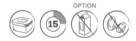

**MAKES** about ½ cup (1 tablespoon per serving)
**PREP TIME:** 3 minutes  |  **COOK TIME:** 6 minutes

**5½ tablespoons unsalted butter or ghee**

**2 tablespoons plus 2 teaspoons water**

**5½ tablespoons powdered sweetener**

**1½ teaspoons vanilla extract**

**¾ teaspoon maple extract**

**⅛ teaspoon salt**

**3 drops liquid sweetener, or to taste**

1.  Melt the butter in a small saucepan over low heat. Whisk in the water and powdered sweetener and simmer for 3 to 4 minutes. Remove from the heat and stir in the extracts, salt, and liquid sweetener.

2.  The syrup will thicken as it cools, and it may separate and crystallize. Be sure to whisk it well; using an immersion blender helps keep it blended. Serve warm and stir before serving.

**WAFFLE ONLY:**
Calories: 158 | Fat: 12.8g | Protein: 8.3g | Carbs: 2.2g | Fiber: 0.4g | Erythritol: 8g

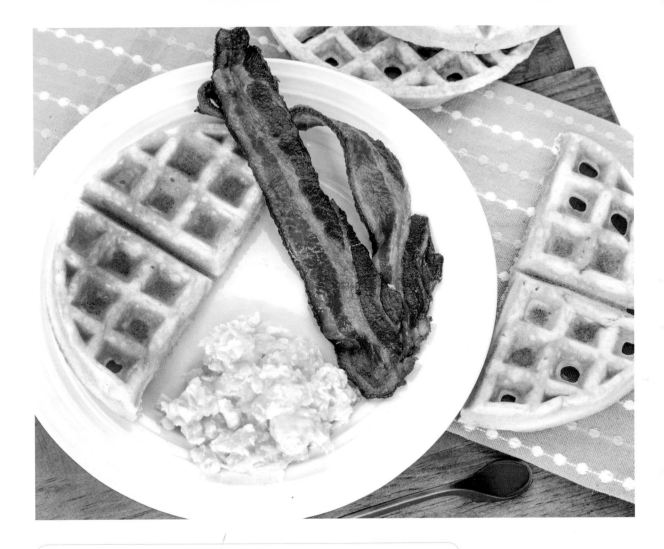

**Cook's Notes:** If you're making these waffles to use as buns for breakfast sandwiches (see page 27), omit the sweetener and add ¼ teaspoon of a savory spice such as garlic or onion powder, if you wish. The savory version makes a great breakfast sandwich and allows you to avoid sweeteners. If, on the other hand, you like sweet and salty combinations, like I do, then you can leave the sweetener in the batter and fill your sandwich with salty bacon or ham.

**Crazy Busy Kitchen Tip:** Make a double batch of waffles on the weekend and freeze them if you won't use them within a week. They are perfect pulled straight from the freezer and toasted in a toaster or in a skillet with some butter. We also have traveled with them, topping them with peanut butter or using them for breakfast sandwiches.

**Crazy Busy Travel Tip:** Take premade waffles on the road with you. Use them as a stand-in for the conventional waffles available at a continental breakfast buffet or as the "buns" for a keto breakfast sandwich (see above). For easy-to-find sandwich fillings, cream cheese is a good bet. (Any place that offers a continental breakfast buffet is likely to serve bagels and cream cheese.) Add precooked bacon or hard-boiled egg slices to your sandwich and you have a perfect meal for traveling!

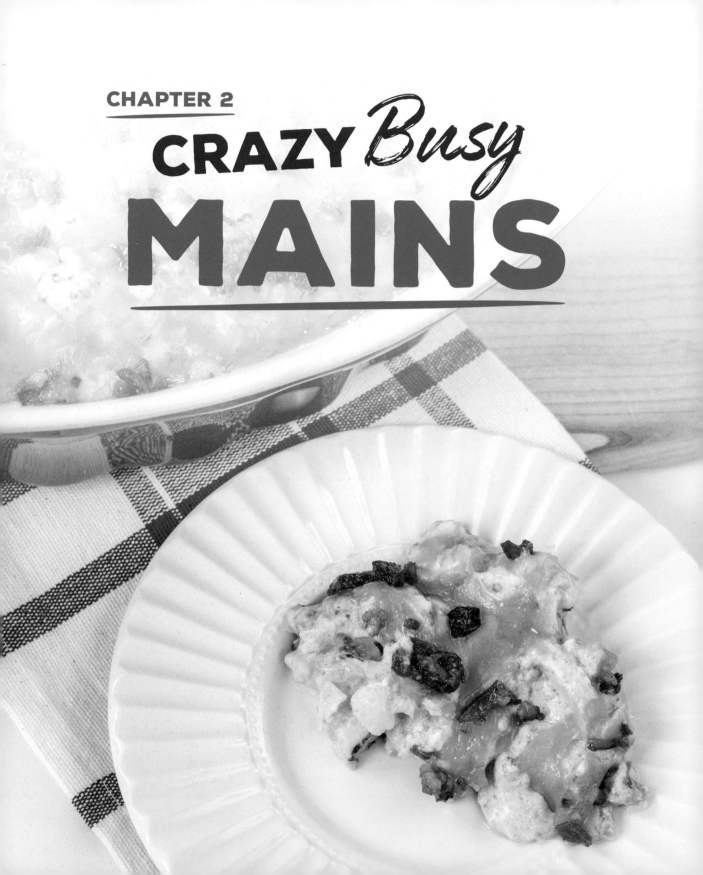

# CHAPTER 2
# CRAZY Busy
# MAINS

"What do we have to eat?" is rarely asked twenty-four hours in advance. Instead, it's one of those questions that gives you less than a thirty-second head start, especially if the person asking is already rummaging through the fridge. For those times, I've included a few simple main meal ideas that you can either keep stocked or grab without slowing down. These include meal ideas that noncooks, like kids and spouses, can put together themselves.

The recipes in this chapter are primarily designed to be full meals with adequate protein, satiating fat, and minimal carbs. With few exceptions, these recipes don't need sides because they include vegetables. My favorites are the Deconstructed Chicken Cordon Bleu, the Easy Chicken and Beef Enchilada Bake, and the Nachos Two Ways.

Because some of us travel frequently and need meals that can be prepared without a lot of equipment, I've included a few options that can be mixed up without a microwave, cooktop, or oven. These meals can be made with simple tools like a knife, plate, cup or bowl, and basic flatware. Doesn't that make you want to try the Chipotle Chicken Salad, the Cold Tossed Pizza Bowl, and the Shrimp Salad–Stuffed Avocado Boats?

If you only have access to a microwave—for example, if you live in a dorm, use a workroom kitchen, or have a hotel stay—you can still enjoy a complete hot or cold keto meal. How about 5-Minute Lasagna, Buffalo Chicken Bake with Bacon and Ranch, or Thai Chicken Slaw with Peanut Sauce? Later in the book, I even show you how to make a cheesecake in the microwave! (See page 144.)

For when you have a little more time, this chapter also includes some great recipes that you can prep in advance and warm up for a family dinner or an individual meal. Many of these favorites make great lunches, too. The Individual BBQ Chicken Pizzas are one example.

Main dishes on keto are easy to create when you focus on a source of protein, add fat for nutrition and flavor, and then choose ingredients that round out the meal while keeping carbs in check.

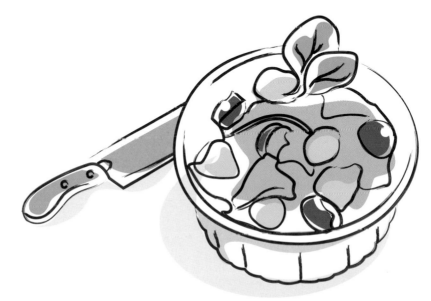

# MEAL *Ideas*

## LOW-CARB FREEZER PIZZAS

Make personal-sized Shortcut Pizza Crusts, then par-bake them and freeze them for fast future meals. To make the crusts, complete Steps 1 and 2 on page 56. When ready to use, defrost as many crusts as you'd like, and then top them with sauce and your favorite pizza toppings. Bake at 375°F for 12 to 15 minutes, or until the crust is warm and lightly browned and the cheese, if used, is bubbly and lightly browned. These crusts thaw quickly, but if you don't have time to let them thaw completely, they are thin enough to use frozen. You may have to bake the pizza for an additional 5 to 8 minutes. Keep a close watch on it so that the toppings don't burn, and make sure that the crust is warmed through before serving. Using a lower oven rack can help.

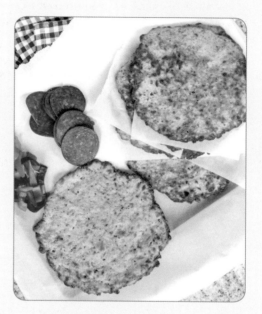

## BLT WRAPS

BLT wraps are just more evidence that the simplest meal ideas can be the tastiest. This is my default lunch. If you use precooked bacon, BLT wraps are easy to make even when you don't have access to a kitchen. The recipe calls for a dollop of mayonnaise on each wrap, but ranch dressing is equally delicious. I like to serve these wraps with homemade or store-bought cheese crisps, which provide a little crunch that reminds me of chips and make this feel a bit more like a meal. To make the wraps, wash and pat dry 3 large romaine lettuce leaves. Lay each leaf flat on a plate or other clean work surface. Top each leaf with 2 strips of cooked bacon and a slice of tomato. Sprinkle with salt and pepper. Place 2 teaspoons of mayonnaise on top of each tomato slice. Roll up the lettuce leaves to create wraps. Serve immediately or later the same day; these wraps don't keep well for long.

*Crazy Busy Travel Tip:* If traveling, make these wraps with precooked bacon that you prepared in advance or buy packaged precooked bacon at the store. You can also use grape tomatoes that don't need to be sliced; just remember that each grape tomato has roughly 0.7 gram of carbs. Lastly, you can use travel packs of mayonnaise that don't require refrigeration.

## SIMPLE SALSA VERDE CHICKEN

You can make this meal with no cooking whatsoever! You can even prepare it without a kitchen, so it's ideal when traveling or living in a dorm. When shopping for salsa verde, remember to check the ingredients and to look for brands with the least carbs and the fewest ingredients. (My favorite is Herdez Salsa Verde. It has 1 gram of carbs per 2-tablespoon serving and some of the same ingredients that I would use in homemade salsa verde.) I prefer to simmer the chicken in the salsa so that the ingredients become warm and the salsa thickens, but doing so is completely optional; this meal is also good served cold.

To make, warm prepared salsa verde in a skillet over medium-low heat. Add cubed or shredded cooked chicken or cooked chicken breast tenderloins and simmer until thoroughly warmed. Top the chicken with fresh or premade guacamole, sour cream, and/or shredded cheese to add fat and flavor to the meal. You can top it with chopped fresh cilantro as well. Serve immediately. Store leftovers in the refrigerator for up to 4 days.

> *Note:* A good ratio of salsa to meat is 1 cup of salsa to 1 pound of cooked chicken. This quantity of meat will serve four people.

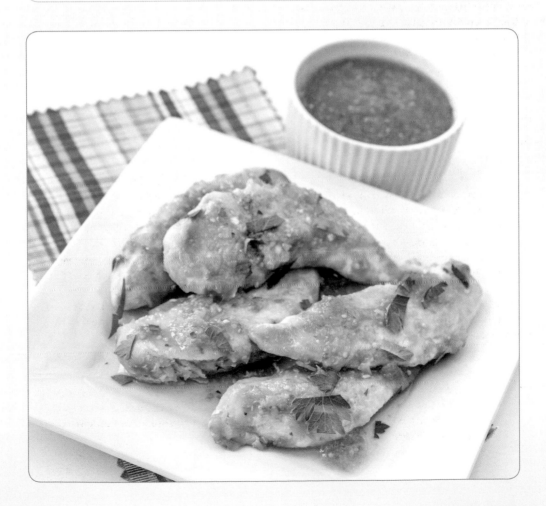

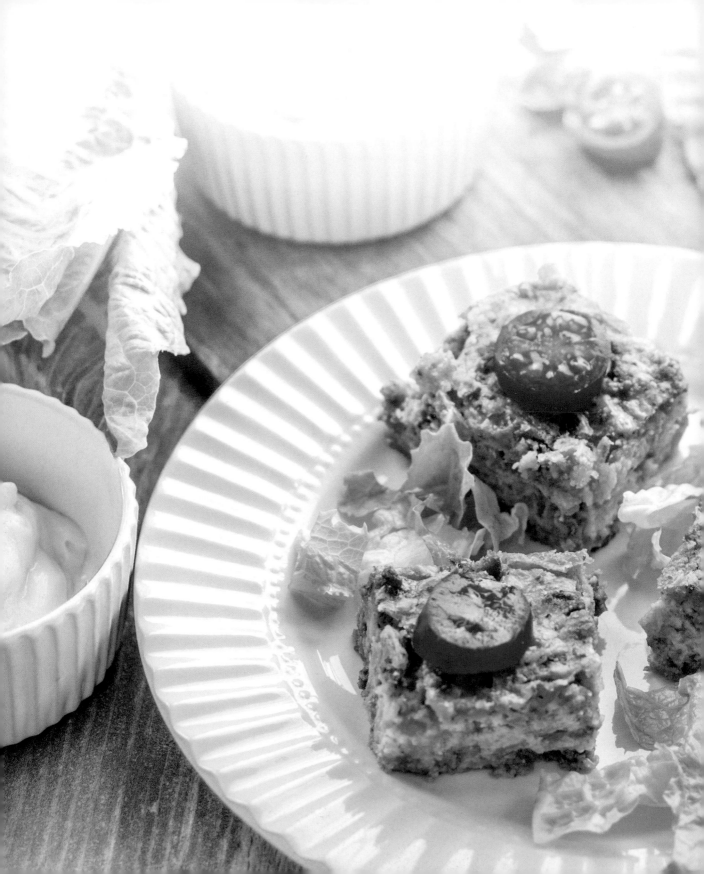

# Recipes

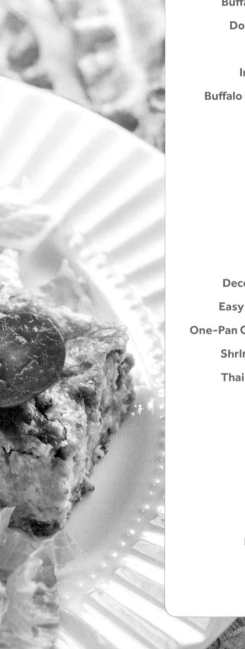

# BUFFALO CHICKEN RANCH NO-TATO SALAD

**MAKES** 6 servings | **PREP TIME:** 8 minutes, plus 1 hour to chill (not including time to cook chicken or bacon if not purchased precooked)

*You will not miss the potatoes in this recipe! Although potato salad is traditionally a side dish, adding chicken gives it the right to take center stage and makes it the perfect hearty one-dish meal. Not only is this cold salad perfect for an easy summer lunch, but it's also a quick dish to take along for a day at the lake or to share at a potluck.*

*You can also make this dish using radishes instead of cauliflower. When I substitute radishes, I like to slice or dice them and then steam them in a skillet. Then I cook off the water and lightly pan-fry the radishes in a little butter until tender. Let them cool before adding them to the bowl with the chicken and bacon.*

**2 (12-ounce) bags frozen cauliflower florets, cooked, drained, and chopped into bite-sized pieces**

**4 cups shredded cooked chicken (about 1 pound)**

**¾ cup crumbled cooked bacon (about 12 strips)**

**1 cup mayonnaise**

**⅓ cup Buffalo wing sauce**

**¼ cup sour cream**

**1 tablespoon lemon juice**

**2 tablespoons ranch seasoning mix**

**4 ounces cheddar cheese, shredded, or 4 ounces blue cheese, crumbled (about 1 cup)**

**3 green onions, sliced**

**¼ teaspoon salt**

**Dash of ground black pepper**

1. Use a clean towel or paper towel to squeeze as much moisture as possible from the cauliflower.

2. Put the cauliflower, chicken, and bacon in a large bowl.

3. In a small bowl, whisk together the mayonnaise, Buffalo sauce, sour cream, lemon juice, and ranch seasoning mix until well combined and creamy. Pour the dressing over the chicken mixture and stir to coat.

4. Add the cheese, green onions, salt, and pepper and toss to combine. Refrigerate the salad for at least 1 hour before serving. Store leftovers in the refrigerator for up to 3 days.

Calories: 432 | Fat: 32.9g | Protein: 31.8g | Carbs: 6.2g | Fiber: 2.7g

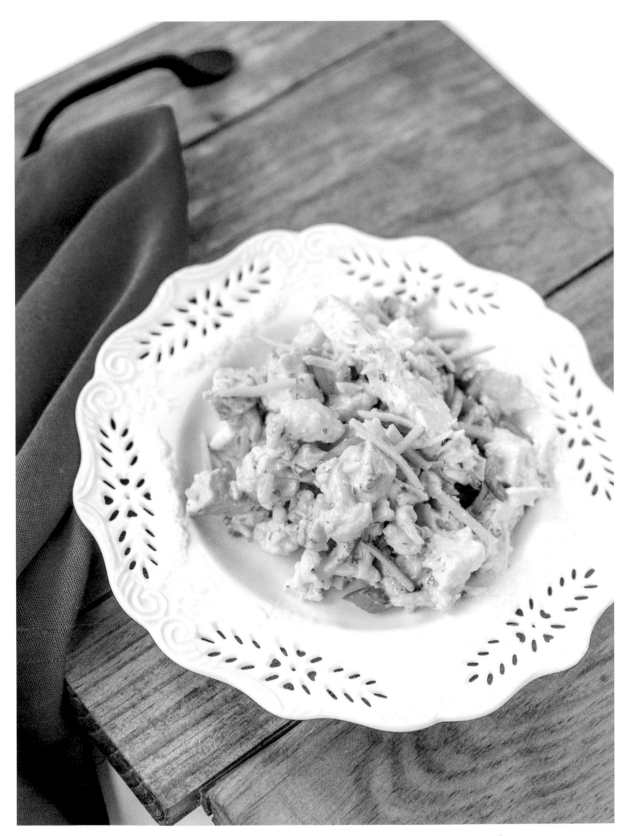

# DOUBLE BACON CHEESEBURGER BAKE

**MAKES** 6 servings  |  **PREP TIME:** 12 minutes (not including time to cook ground beef or bacon if not purchased precooked)  |  **COOK TIME:** 25 minutes

*Combine all the best burger toppings and you get a hearty dish that is easy to make and perfect to serve to a crowd or to provide multiple meals. For portion control, you can bake this in a mini muffin pan or a standard-size muffin pan, which gives a nice crisp finish on the edges. I like to serve it with traditional burger toppings, such as shredded lettuce, sliced red onions, pickles, mustard, mayonnaise, and/or a dollop of ranch dressing.*

6 ounces cream cheese (¾ cup), softened

2 large eggs

½ cup mayonnaise

8 ounces cheddar cheese, shredded (about 2 cups)

½ cup shredded Parmesan cheese

1⅓ ounces mozzarella cheese, shredded (about ⅓ cup)

1 pound ground beef, cooked, crumbled, and drained

¾ cup chopped cooked bacon (about 12 strips)

2 tablespoons dried minced onion

2 teaspoons Worcestershire sauce

1 teaspoon baking powder

1 teaspoon salt

½ teaspoon garlic powder

3 cherry tomatoes, sliced, for serving (optional)

1.  Preheat the oven to 375°F. Grease a 9 by 13-inch baking dish.

2.  In a large bowl, beat the cream cheese and eggs until creamy. Add the mayonnaise and cheeses and stir to combine. Stir in the cooked ground beef, bacon, dried minced onion, Worcestershire sauce, baking powder, salt, and garlic powder until well combined. Pour the mixture into the prepared baking dish.

3.  Bake for 25 to 30 minutes, or until browned and bubbly. Let cool for 5 to 10 minutes before slicing and serving. Garnish each portion with a cherry tomato slice, if desired. Store leftovers in the refrigerator for up to 4 days or freeze for up to 2 months.

*Crazy Busy Kitchen Tip:* Use precooked bacon and leftover burgers to make this recipe. Just crumble the cooked burgers and prepare the recipe as directed. If you don't have a full pound of leftover hamburgers, you can cut the recipe in half or freeze crumbled hamburgers until you have enough to make a full batch.

Calories: 667 | Fat: 35g | Protein: 31g | Carbs: 4.8g | Fiber: 2.4g

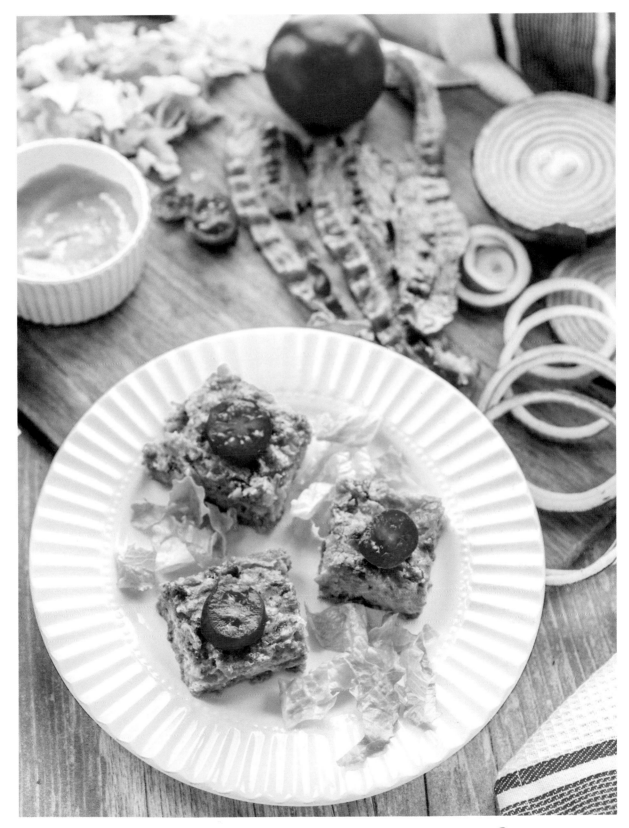

# 5-MINUTE LASAGNA

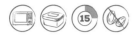

**MAKES** 2 servings | **PREP TIME:** 2 minutes, plus 5 minutes to cool (not including time to cook sausage if not purchased precooked) | **COOK TIME:** 3 minutes

*Using store-bought precooked sausage or leftover cooked sausage, or browning the sausage ahead of time, makes this a really quick meal. My kids can assemble it themselves, or I can prep it in advance and they can microwave it when they are hungry. This is a perfect meal for those hectic weeknights when we all eat at different times. The ingredients are simple, inexpensive, and generally kept stocked in our kitchen. The hardest part about making this delicious dish is waiting for it to cool!*

¼ cup full-fat ricotta cheese

⅓ cup chopped pepperoni

¼ cup cooked and crumbled Italian sausage

2 ounces mozzarella cheese, shredded (about ½ cup)

½ cup tomato sauce

½ teaspoon Italian seasoning

⅛ teaspoon garlic powder

**1.** Divide the ricotta evenly between two microwave-safe 8-ounce ramekins. Top each with half of the pepperoni and half of the sausage. Sprinkle one-quarter of the mozzarella (about 2 tablespoons) into each ramekin, then pour ¼ cup of tomato sauce into each dish. Sprinkle the Italian seasoning and garlic powder into the ramekins. Top with the remaining ¼ cup of mozzarella.

**2.** Microwave at full power for 45 seconds to 1 minute, or until the cheese is melted and the lasagna is bubbling. Watch carefully, as microwave cooking times vary. You may want to use two 45-second increments of cooking time.

**3.** Use a dish towel or oven mitt to remove the ramekins from the microwave. Let the lasagna cool for 5 to 10 minutes before serving.

*Cook's Notes:* No ramekins? No time to shop for some? No problem! You can also use small cereal bowls or extra-large coffee mugs. Just make sure they are microwave-safe.

My microwave has 1250 watts. If yours has a lower wattage, you may need to increase the cooking time a bit.

*Crazy Busy Shopping Tip:* Look for the ricotta with the highest fat content and lowest carb count. Store brands are often the best option. Also, one 8-ounce can of tomato sauce is perfect for a double batch of this recipe (four servings). Many brands cost only about a quarter per can.

*Crazy Busy Kitchen Tip:* This dish can be assembled, refrigerated, and cooked later.

**Variation: Oven-Baked Lasagna.** The lasagna can be baked at 350°F for 10 to 12 minutes, or until bubbling and lightly browned.

Calories: 331 | Fat: 25.2g | Protein: 20.1g | Carbs: 2.2g | Fiber: 1g

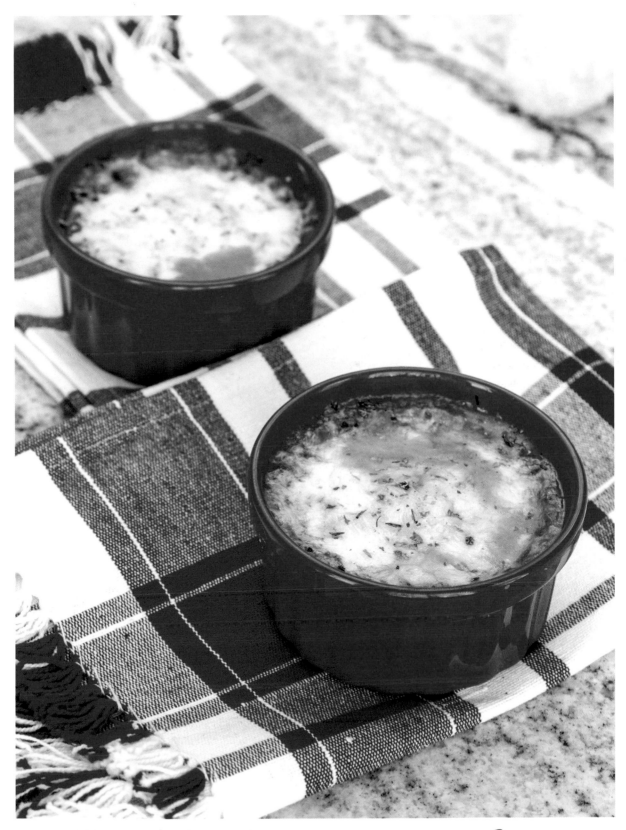

# INDIVIDUAL BBQ CHICKEN PIZZAS

**(30)** | **MAKES** 1 to 6 servings | **PREP TIME:** 4 minutes (not including time to cook chicken if not purchased precooked) | **COOK TIME:** 26 minutes

*While you can easily use this quantity of dough to make one large pizza (see the variation at right), I usually form it into six individual-sized crusts that I par-bake and stick in the freezer for quick and easy meals later (see the Meal Idea on page 46). In fact, while pizzas made with par-baked crusts are one of my Plan B meals, they're tasty enough to be part of a meal plan as well. This meal plan concept is easy because it uses items you're likely to find in your pantry. It's quick because once you've par-baked the crusts, all you need to do is to top them and pop them in the oven. By the time you've cleared a place at the table, poured a glass of water, and fed the dog, your pizza is delivered—fresh, hot, and low-carb! In this recipe, I walk you through the process of forming the dough into individual pizza crusts and give the topping quantities for one pizza so that you can easily make one or more small pizzas and freeze the remaining par-baked crusts for later. Barbecue chicken is one of my family's absolute favorite toppings, but feel free to use more traditional toppings such as mozzarella, sausage, or pepperoni, if you prefer. My shortcut pizza crust is great topped with just about anything!*

## SHORTCUT PIZZA CRUST(S):

*(Makes six 5½-inch round crusts or one 10 by 16-inch rectangular crust)*

**6 ounces mozzarella cheese, shredded (about 1½ cups)**

**2 tablespoons cream cheese, softened**

**1 large egg**

**⅓ cup blanched almond flour**

**⅓ cup oat fiber (or use an additional ⅓ cup almond flour)**

**1 teaspoon baking powder**

**1 teaspoon garlic salt**

**1 teaspoon Italian seasoning**

## BBQ CHICKEN TOPPING FOR ONE *(for one 5½-inch crust):*

**2 tablespoons sugar-free BBQ sauce**

**2 tablespoons shredded smoked Gouda or cheddar cheese**

**A handful of red onion slices**

**4 ounces chopped cooked chicken**

**2 ounces mozzarella cheese, shredded (about ½ cup)**

1. Preheat the oven to 350°F. Line an 11 by 17-inch or larger baking sheet with parchment paper and lightly grease the parchment.

2. Put all the ingredients for the crust in a stand mixer, or use a mixing bowl and hand mixer, and blend into a dough. It will be slightly sticky. Divide the dough into 6 equal portions, moistening your hands lightly with water or oil as needed to keep the dough from sticking. Press each portion into a 5-inch round crust and place on the prepared baking sheet at least 1 inch apart to allow for spreading. Par-bake for 14 to 16 minutes, or until lightly browned. Remove the crusts from the oven. If reserving the crusts for later, transfer them to a cooling rack. When cool, stack, separated with sheets of parchment paper, and freeze in a freezer-safe bag for up to 3 months.

3. To make an individual-sized BBQ Chicken Pizza, increase the oven temperature to 375°F.

4. Spread the BBQ sauce over one par-baked crust. Sprinkle the Gouda on top of the sauce. Spread the onion slices and chicken evenly over the cheese. Top with the mozzarella. Bake for 12 to 15 minutes, or until the cheeses are melted and lightly browned.

**Air fryer instructions:** Place the topped individual-sized pizza on the rack in an air fryer. Cook on high for 8 to 9 minutes, or until the cheeses are melted and lightly browned.

### SHORTCUT PIZZA CRUST ONLY:

Calories: 144 | Fat: 10.3g | Protein: 9.8g | Carbs: 2.3g | Fiber: 0.7g

### BBQ CHICKEN TOPPING:

Calories: 275 | Fat: 15.1g | Protein: 21.8g | Carbs: 2.7g | Fiber: 0g

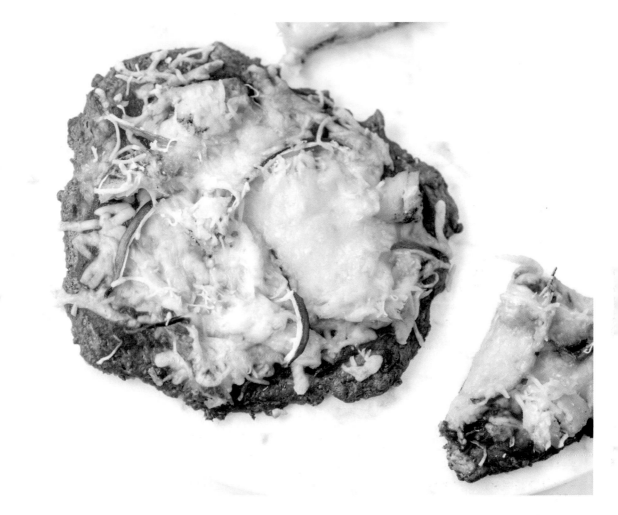

**Variation: Large BBQ Chicken Pizza for Six.** To make one large pizza, dump the dough onto the prepared baking sheet and use your hands to press the dough into a rectangle, about 10 by 16 inches. Create a raised edge around the sides. Spread ½ cup of BBQ sauce over the crust. Sprinkle ¾ cup (about 3 ounces) of shredded smoked Gouda or cheddar cheese on top of the sauce. Next, spread about ⅓ scant cup of red onion slices and 1½ pounds of chopped cooked chicken evenly across the crust. Top with 3 cups of shredded mozzarella cheese (about 12 ounces). Bake at 375°F for 18 to 20 minutes, or until the cheeses are melted and lightly browned.

*Cook's Notes:* This pizza dough is based on the famous fathead dough, which is easy to make and delicious but isn't always fast. The original recipe calls for melting the cheeses and then adding the other ingredients. In the meantime, the dough can become stringy, sticky, and difficult to work with. In this shortcut version, you mix all the ingredients together in a stand mixer (or use a bowl and hand mixer). Once you have a "dough," shaping the crusts is relatively easy.

*Crazy Busy Shopping Tip:* Look for sugar-free BBQ sauce sweetened with stevia, erythritol, monk fruit, or xylitol. It's best to avoid anything with sugars such as molasses or corn syrup. I like Stevia Sweet brand.

*Crazy Busy Kitchen Tip:* Use leftover chicken, canned chicken, or rotisserie chicken to make this recipe really fast and economical.

# BUFFALO CHICKEN BAKE WITH BACON AND RANCH

**MAKES** 6 servings | **PREP TIME:** 10 minutes (not including time to cook chicken or bacon if not purchased precooked, or to cook cauliflower) | **COOK TIME:** 24 minutes

*So much yum! Just look at the ingredients, and you will see that this recipe is packed with flavor. You can skip the blue cheese if you don't love it, and you can use store-bought precooked bacon if you don't have any already made.*

1 (8-ounce) package cream cheese, softened

⅓ cup sour cream

⅓ cup Buffalo wing sauce

⅓ cup ranch dressing, plus more for serving if desired

4 cups shredded cooked chicken

2 medium stalks celery, chopped (about ⅔ cup), plus more celery sticks for serving if desired

2 tablespoons dried minced onion

1 teaspoon garlic powder

8 ounces shredded cheddar cheese (about 2 cups), divided

1 (12-ounce) package frozen cauliflower florets, cooked and drained

4 ounces blue cheese or cheddar cheese, crumbled or shredded (about 1 cup)

½ cup cooked bacon pieces

1. Preheat the oven to 350°F. Grease a 9 by 13-inch baking dish.

2. In a large bowl, mix together the cream cheese, sour cream, Buffalo sauce, and ranch dressing until well blended and creamy. Stir in the chicken, celery, dried minced onion, garlic powder, and half of the cheddar cheese.

3. Use a clean kitchen towel or paper towel to squeeze the moisture from the cooked cauliflower, then chop the florets into bite-sized pieces. Add the cauliflower to the chicken mixture and stir well.

4. Spread the chicken mixture in the prepared baking dish. Sprinkle the blue cheese crumbles, the remaining 1 cup of cheddar cheese, and the bacon pieces evenly over the top of the casserole.

5. Bake for 24 to 28 minutes, or until bubbly. The cheese topping should be melted and lightly browned. Serve warm with extra ranch dressing and celery sticks, if desired. Store leftovers in the refrigerator for up to 4 days.

*Crazy Busy Kitchen Tip:* Make it faster by using canned or rotisserie chicken. Grab the celery from the grocery store salad bar. You need only two stalks for this recipe (plus some additional stalks for serving, if desired), and unless you know you will use celery at another meal, you can easily grab ⅔ cup of celery (the rough equivalent of two medium stalks) for less than $1. Not only will you save money, but the celery from the salad bar is already washed and chopped, saving you additional time!

Calories: 588 | Fat: 37.2g | Protein: 33.1g | Carbs: 4.7g | Fiber: 1.9g

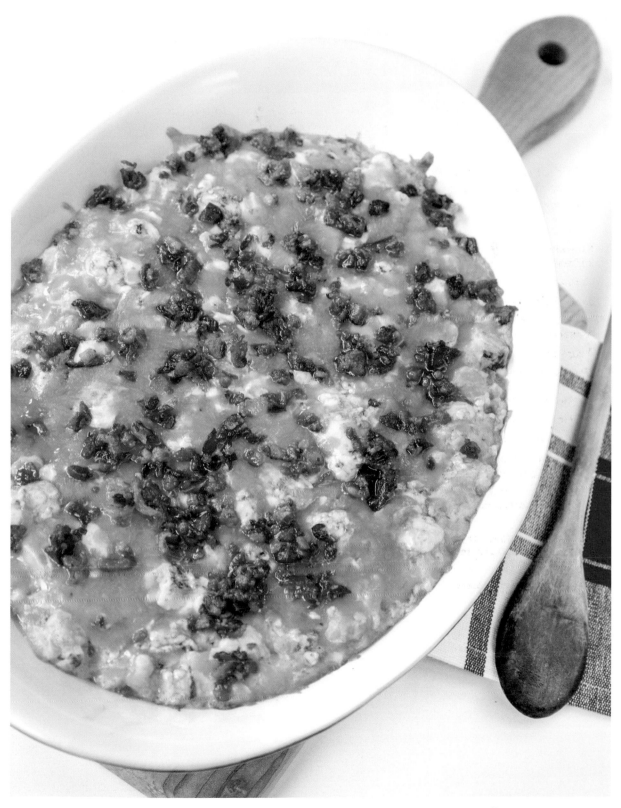

# NACHOS TWO WAYS

**MAKES** 4 servings | **PREP TIME:** 10 minutes (not including time to cook chicken or brown ground beef if not purchased precooked) | **COOK TIME:** 10 minutes

*I love this recipe because nachos can be as simple or complex as you choose to make them. In this recipe, I give you two main meat options: chicken or beef. You can add whatever fresh toppings you have on hand—chopped tomatoes, fresh jalapeños, bell peppers, or poblanos are excellent additions if you have them. If you don't have fresh toppings, this recipe can be made with entirely shelf-stable ingredients, including canned chicken, ground beef, or even pulled pork, which makes it perfect for Crazy Busy Keto.*

**SEASONED MEAT:**

1 pound chopped cooked chicken, or 1 pound ground beef, cooked, crumbled, and drained

2 teaspoons ground cumin

1½ teaspoons chili powder

1 teaspoon garlic powder

1 teaspoon onion powder

¼ teaspoon salt

2 tablespoons salted butter

2 tablespoons water

2 cups shredded lettuce

1⅓ cups Parmesan cheese crisps

1 cup Mexican Fiesta Cauli Rice (page 124) (optional)

4 ounces cheddar cheese, shredded (about 1 cup)

½ cup sour cream

**OPTIONAL TOPPINGS:**

½ cup prepared enchilada sauce

1 (4-ounce) can diced green chilies, drained

2 tablespoons chopped pickled jalapeños

2 tablespoons chopped fresh cilantro

1. In a large skillet over medium heat, toss the cooked chicken or beef with the spices, salt, butter, and water until the chicken is coated with the seasonings. Cook, stirring occasionally, until everything is warmed through. Set aside.

2. Divide the lettuce among four plates. Top each plate with equal amounts of the cheese crisps, cauli rice (if using), seasoned meat, cheese, sour cream, and any additional toppings you like. Serve immediately.

3. Store leftover prepared chicken or ground beef separately from the other ingredients so that you can warm the meat and create a fresh nacho platter for a later meal. The ingredients will keep in the refrigerator for up to 4 days.

*Crazy Busy Kitchen Tip:* Use bagged preshredded lettuce if you don't have time to wash and shred your own. If you're making only one or two servings of nachos, you may want to get the cheese and jalapeños from the grocery store salad bar. Diced tomatoes and bell peppers are other good nacho toppings to buy from the salad bar.

Calories: 546 | Fat: 34.3g | Protein: 28.9g | Carbs: 4.2g | Fiber: 1.6g

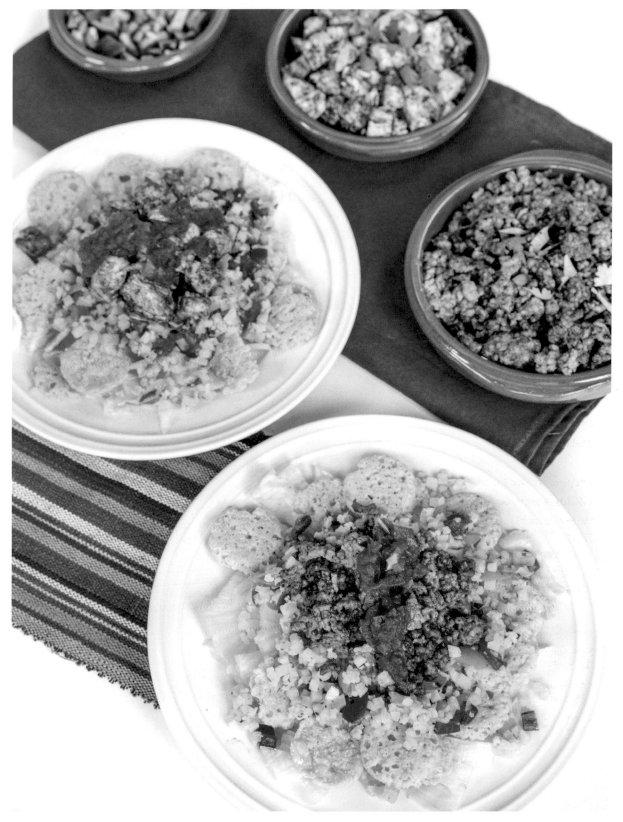

# CHICKEN À LA KING

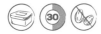

**MAKES** 4 servings | **PREP TIME:** 4 minutes (not including time to cook chicken if not purchased precooked) | **COOK TIME:** 18 minutes

*Chicken à la king was a very popular dish from about the 1950s until the late 1970s. By the '80s, it had become too commonplace to be worthy of royalty. Although I hadn't had it since I was a child, I remembered it one day as having a fatty sauce that would be easy to make low-carb. This version uses chicken broth and powdered bone broth, a great keto-friendly substitute for bouillon. The bone broth powder enriches the flavor without adding more liquid so that the sauce is thicker. Another trick for thickening the sauce is to incorporate egg yolks. Adding tempered egg yolks over low heat creates a thick, rich gravy similar to hollandaise. You can omit them, but this dish is much better with the yolks. The sherry is optional as well, but it gives the sauce a signature flavor.*

**6 tablespoons (¾ stick) salted butter**

**8 ounces mushrooms, sliced**

**1 medium stalk celery, chopped (about ⅓ cup)**

**⅓ cup chopped bell peppers or mini sweet peppers (any color)**

**¼ cup chopped onions**

**1 cup heavy cream**

**½ cup chicken broth**

**2 ounces cream cheese (¼ cup)**

**1 ounce jarred diced pimentos, drained**

**1 tablespoon powdered chicken bone broth (see Tip)**

**2 tablespoons cooking sherry (optional)**

**2 large egg yolks, room temperature, beaten**

**5 cups shredded or chopped cooked chicken, warmed in the microwave**

**¼ teaspoon salt**

**⅛ teaspoon ground white pepper**

1. Melt the butter in a large skillet over medium heat. Add the mushrooms, celery, bell peppers, and onions, increase the heat to medium-high, and sauté the veggies until just tender, 5 to 7 minutes.

2. Reduce the heat to medium-low and add the heavy cream, broth, cream cheese, pimentos, and powdered bone broth, if using. Stir to melt the cream cheese and bone broth powder. Simmer for an additional 6 to 8 minutes, or until the sauce is reduced by half. Remove the pan from the heat and stir in the sherry, if using.

3. In a small bowl, whisk 3 tablespoons of the hot sauce into the egg yolks. Slowly pour the tempered yolks into the skillet with the veggies and sauce, stirring continuously.

4. Add the chicken, salt, and pepper to the skillet and stir to incorporate it into the sauce mixture. Return the pan to low heat if needed to thoroughly warm the dish, taking care to keep the heat low so that the eggs don't curdle. Serve immediately.

*Crazy Busy Shopping Tips:* Use rotisserie chicken and the grocery store salad bar to make this recipe easier and faster. You can grab the celery, bell peppers, and onions already prepped from the salad bar!

*Powdered bone broth adds a rich flavor but isn't required. I use this Ketologie brand product, labeled "Bone Broth Powdered Drink Mix," as a bouillon substitute. In an ideal world, a keto-friendly bouillon option would be readily available, but I've searched high and low and cannot find one. If you do, feel free to use it in place of the powdered bone broth.*

Calories: 643 | Fat: 56g | Protein: 32g | Carbs: 5.4g | Fiber: 0.7g

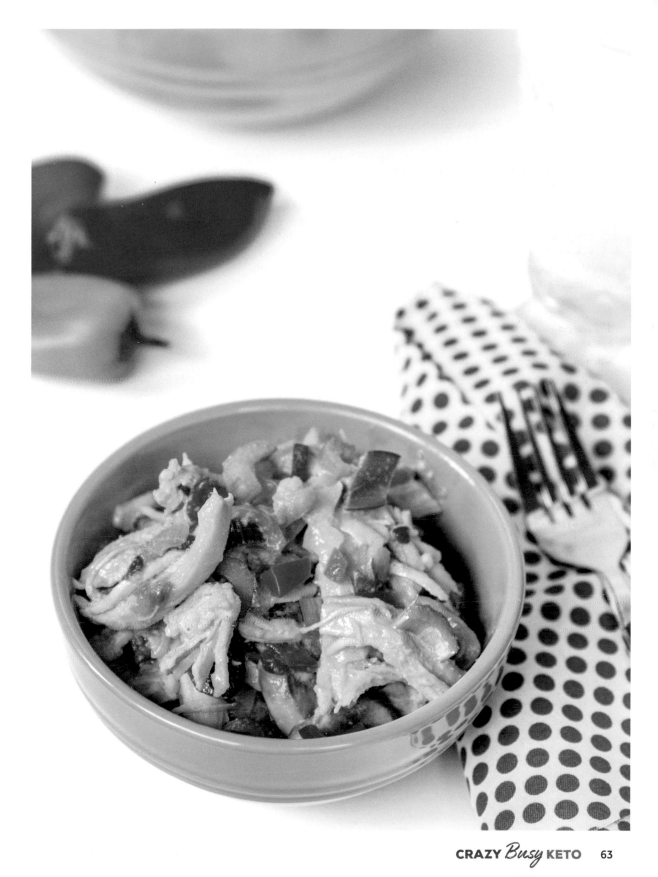

# CHILE RELLENOS CASSEROLE

**MAKES** 8 servings | **PREP TIME:** 5 minutes, plus 10 minutes to cool (not including time to cook chicken if not purchased precooked) | **COOK TIME:** 30 minutes

*My husband spied me putting this dish together and said, "That's a whole lotta cheese!" I took it as a compliment. Unlike the eggy breakfast casserole that you may have tried before, this recipe is much more of a cheesy, creamy casserole without a hint of the egg that helps hold it together. Since this dish takes a bit longer to bake, it's perfect to make ahead of time. This is one of those meals that you can put together while you're already in the kitchen cooking. It can bake while you eat and clean the kitchen. Once it cools, you can portion it into future lunch or dinner servings and refrigerate them.*

**4 cups chopped cooked chicken, divided**

**4 (7-ounce) cans whole green chilies, drained, divided**

**2 tablespoons dried minced onion, divided**

**8 ounces cheddar cheese, shredded (about 2 cups), divided**

**8 ounces Monterey Jack cheese, shredded (about 2 cups), divided**

**2 ounces Cotija cheese, crumbled (about ½ cup), divided (optional)**

**¾ cup heavy cream**

**2 large eggs**

**½ teaspoon garlic powder**

**½ teaspoon baking powder**

**¼ teaspoon salt**

**FOR SERVING (OPTIONAL):**

**Prepared enchilada sauce**

**Diced avocado**

**Sour cream**

**Chopped fresh cilantro, for garnish (optional)**

1.  Preheat the oven to 350°F.

2.  Spread half of the cooked chicken in a 9-inch square (or 8 by 12-inch) baking dish. Cover the chicken with a layer of two cans of the drained chilies, 1 tablespoon of the dried minced onion, and half of the cheeses. Repeat the layers with the remaining chicken, chilies, dried minced onion, and cheeses. Set aside.

3.  Use a blender or whisk to whip the cream, eggs, garlic powder, baking powder, and salt. Slowly pour the cream mixture over the entire contents of the baking dish. Use a knife or fork to make sure that the cream mixture saturates the layers.

4.  Bake for 30 to 40 minutes, or until the center is just set. Remove from the oven and let cool for 10 to 15 minutes before serving.

5.  Serve with prepared enchilada sauce, diced avocado, and/or a dollop of sour cream and garnish with fresh cilantro, if desired. Store leftovers in the refrigerator for up to 4 days.

*Cook's Notes:* Add some cooked and crumbled Mexican chorizo to the chicken layer for extra flavor! You could also use a spicy shredded cheese in place of the cheddar or Monterey Jack.

Calories: 499 | Fat: 32.7g | Protein: 33.4g | Carbs: 4.1g | Fiber: 0.7g

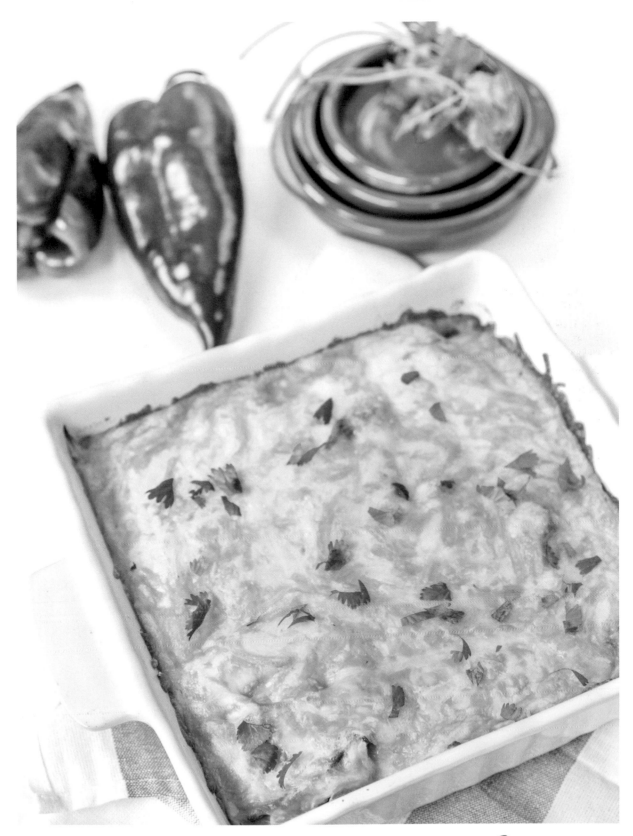

# BAKED CHICKEN PARMESAN

**MAKES** 8 servings
**PREP TIME:** 15 minutes  |  **COOK TIME:** 30 minutes

*Every time I make this recipe, my husband questions my use of crushed tomatoes instead of marinara sauce. You can use either, but I really prefer the chunky pieces of tomatoes. The best part is that when you make the dish this way, the seasoned chicken tenderloins don't require a separate egg wash. This recipe provides just enough "breading" to resemble the high-carb classic.*

**2 pounds chicken breast tenderloins, patted dry**

**⅓ cup mayonnaise**

**Dash of salt**

**Dash of ground black pepper**

**1½ teaspoons Italian seasoning, divided**

**1 teaspoon garlic powder**

**½ cup pork rind dust**

**½ cup shredded Parmesan cheese**

**1 (14.5-ounce) can crushed tomatoes or prepared marinara sauce**

**4 ounces mozzarella cheese, shredded (about 2 cups)**

1. Preheat the oven to 350°F. Line a rimmed baking sheet with parchment paper.

2. Place the chicken in a single layer on the lined baking sheet. Spread the mayonnaise over each piece of chicken and season with the salt and pepper. Sprinkle ½ teaspoon of the Italian seasoning and the garlic powder over the chicken. Top with the pork rind dust and Parmesan cheese.

3. Bake for 20 to 25 minutes, or until the chicken is tender and the pork rind and Parmesan cheese coating is browned and crispy.

4. Remove from the oven, transfer the chicken to a 9 by 13-inch baking dish, and top with the crushed tomatoes. Sprinkle the remaining 1 teaspoon of Italian seasoning over the tomatoes and top with the mozzarella cheese.

5. Return the chicken to the oven and bake for 10 to 15 minutes, or until the cheese is melted and just browned. Serve immediately. Store leftovers in the refrigerator for up to 5 days.

*Crazy Busy Kitchen Tip:* If you aren't going to eat all of the chicken at once, it's best to store the extras after baking the chicken in Step 3, but before adding the tomatoes and cheese and finishing the dish in the oven. When you are ready to serve the reserved chicken, you can top it with the appropriate amounts of tomatoes and cheese and bake it in a preheated 350°F oven until warm and bubbly.

Calories: 285 | Fat: 22g | Protein: 32.1g | Carbs: 3.2g | Fiber: 0.5g

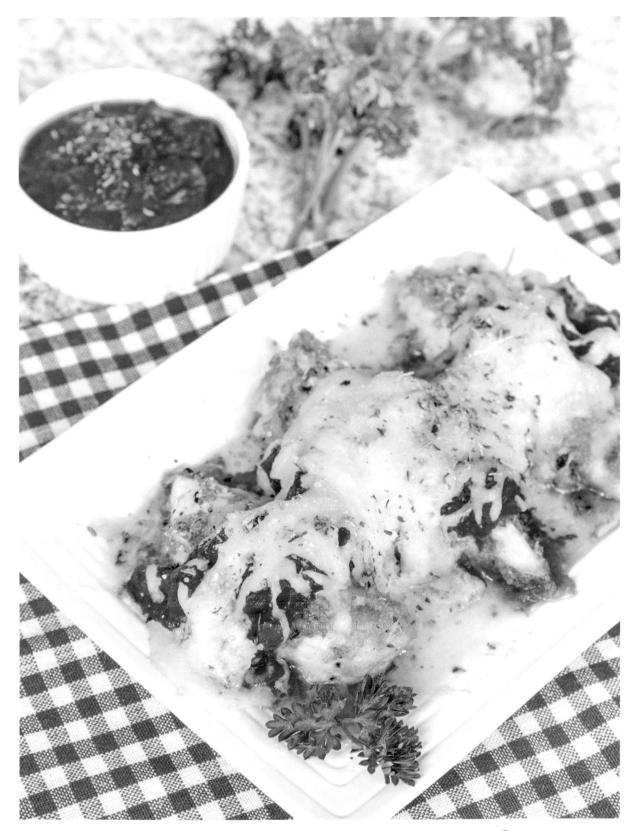

# CHIPOTLE CHICKEN SALAD

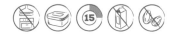

**MAKES** 4 servings | **PREP TIME:** 6 minutes (not including time to cook chicken if not purchased precooked)

*If you adore heat, two chipotle peppers in this chicken salad will not be enough for you. If you're a bit of a lightweight when it comes to spicy food, then one chipotle may be plenty. I compromise and use two and then serve an extra bit of chopped chipotles on the side. If I have it on hand, I also love to add fresh cilantro to this easy chicken salad. This is another dish that seems to taste best the day after it's made, which makes it perfect to prep ahead of time.*

**2 cups chopped cooked chicken**

**½ cup mayonnaise**

**¼ cup chopped celery**

**3 tablespoons lime juice**

**2 tablespoons finely chopped red onions, or 2 teaspoons dried minced onion**

**2 chipotle peppers in adobo sauce, chopped**

**½ teaspoon garlic powder**

**⅛ teaspoon salt**

**½ teaspoon paprika (optional)**

Place all the ingredients except the paprika in a mixing bowl and stir to combine. Sprinkle with the paprika before serving, if desired. This salad is best if refrigerated for at least 30 minutes before eating but can be served immediately if you're in a hurry.

*Crazy Busy Kitchen Tip:* For an even quicker meal, use canned or rotisserie chicken and grab the chopped celery and onions from the grocery store salad bar. Also, instead of hand-chopping the chipotles (my preference for the best flavor and texture), you can toss them into a small blender with the mayo and lime juice and make a quick sauce to pour over the chicken salad.

Calories: 246 | Fat: 38.2g | Protein: 21.3g | Carbs: 3.2g | Fiber: 1.4g

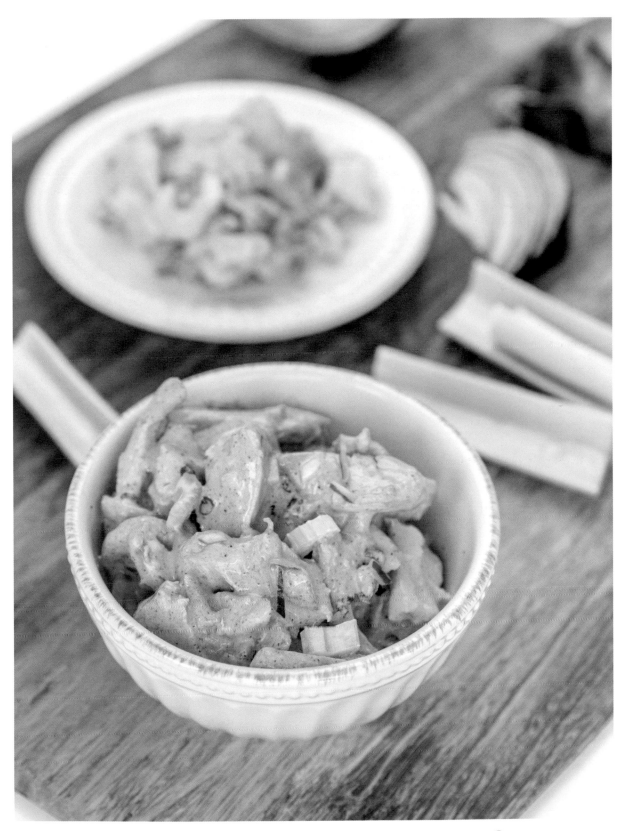

# CHICKEN WINGS THREE WAYS

**MAKES** 4 servings (about 7 wings per person)
**PREP TIME:** 3 to 6 minutes | **COOK TIME:** 30 minutes

*Wings are one of the forbidden foods that you can enjoy guilt-free on a ketogenic diet. Not only are they wonderfully fatty, but they also cook quickly and are easily dressed up with different flavors. In fact, we often cook up a huge batch of wings and have two or three different seasonings waiting. When the wings are hot out of the oven, we toss them with the various seasonings, giving us plenty of tasty options. Three of our favorites are Chili-Lime, Greek, and Traditional Buffalo. I've included all three options for you here, following my basic and foolproof method for crispy, juicy wings.*

**FOR ALL THREE VARIATIONS:**

**2 pounds chicken wings and/or drumettes, trimmed**

**1 teaspoon baking powder**

1. Preheat the oven to 425°F.

2. Pat the chicken dry with a towel to remove as much moisture as possible. Place the chicken wings and/or drumettes in a large bowl, sprinkle them with the baking powder, and toss to coat.

3. Place the wings on a rimmed baking sheet in a single layer. Bake for 30 to 45 minutes, or until the wings are tender and browned. Remove from the oven and let cool for 5 minutes before seasoning according to your preferred variation.

**Calories:** 334 | **Fat:** 22.4g | **Protein:** 24.1g | **Carbs:** 0g | **Fiber:** 0g

# CHILI-LIME WINGS

*Even though I don't typically enjoy spicy foods, the flavor combination of chili and lime is really tasty. The fresh taste of the lime juice brightens the deeper flavor of the chili powder. It just works! And it works really well on chicken wings. Even though David, Grace, and I have different taste preferences for wings, this version is one we can all agree on. We also agree that these wings are great served with ranch dressing—celery optional.*

**1½ tablespoons lime juice**

**1 tablespoon bacon fat, melted, or avocado oil**

**2 tablespoons chili powder**

**1 tablespoon salt**

**2 teaspoons garlic powder**

**Grated zest of 2 limes (optional)**

**2 pounds baked chicken wings and/ or drumettes (from above)**

1. In a large bowl, mix the lime juice and melted bacon fat and set aside. In a small bowl, whisk together the chili powder, salt, garlic powder, and lime zest, if using.

2. Toss the baked wings in the lime juice mixture until each wing is wet. Sprinkle with the dry seasonings and toss to coat. Serve immediately.

**Calories:** 417 | **Fat:** 30.1g | **Protein:** 24.8g | **Carbs:** 1.8g | **Fiber:** 0.7g

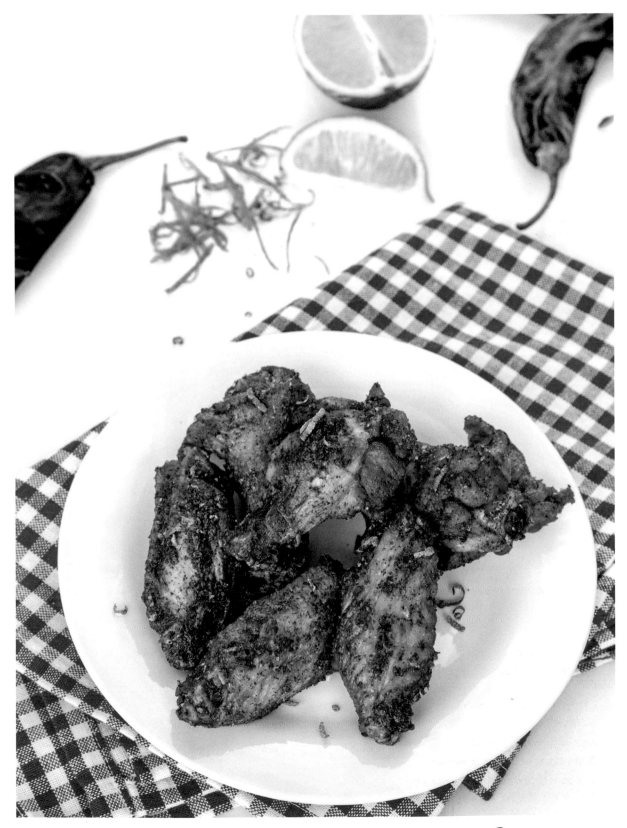

# GREEK WINGS

*I love all things Greek, so the flavors in this recipe are at the top of my list. Subtle hints of lemon and a burst of feta cheese make this a surprising twist on traditional wings. Serve with some Kalamata olives, lemon wedges, and either Tzatziki Sauce (page 132) or Feta Cream Sauce (page 130), and your taste buds will yell, "Opa!"*

2 tablespoons olive oil

Grated zest of 1 lemon

Juice of 1 large lemon (about ¼ cup)

2 teaspoons minced garlic

2 teaspoons ground oregano

1 teaspoon paprika

¼ teaspoon ground black pepper

⅛ teaspoon cayenne pepper (optional)

1 teaspoon salt

2 pounds baked chicken wings and/or drumettes (from page 70)

1 ounce feta cheese, crumbled (about ¼ cup) (omit for dairy-free)

1. In a large bowl, whisk together the olive oil, lemon zest, lemon juice, and garlic. In a smaller bowl, mix together the dried spices and salt.

2. Toss the baked wings in the olive oil mixture. Add the dry seasoning mixture and toss to coat the wings well. Sprinkle the crumbled feta over the wings, if using, and serve immediately.

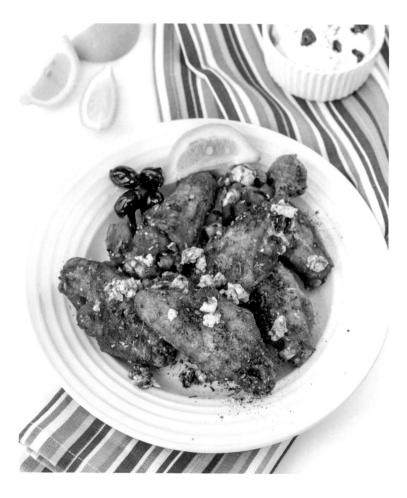

Calories: 423 | Fat: 32.6g | Protein: 25.5g | Carbs: 1.8g | Fiber: 0.7g

# TRADITIONAL BUFFALO WINGS

*Maybe it's boring or maybe it's a classic, but this is my husband's favorite dish by far. I'll call him a traditionalist, lest I get myself into trouble. And if I do get in trouble, I'll just feed him these tried-and-true Buffalo wings! This recipe is super easy and fast if you use store-bought Buffalo wing sauce. Also, these wings are great with the classic accompaniment of blue cheese or ranch dressing. Strict traditionalists will require a celery stick on the plate as well.*

⅓ cup Buffalo wing sauce

2 tablespoons salted butter, melted, or avocado oil

1 tablespoon lemon juice

½ teaspoon minced garlic

2 pounds baked chicken wings and/or drumettes (from page 70)

1 tablespoon chopped fresh cilantro, for garnish (optional)

In a large bowl, whisk together the Buffalo sauce, melted butter, lemon juice, and garlic to make a sauce. Toss the baked wings in the sauce, then serve immediately. Garnish with fresh cilantro, if desired.

*Crazy Busy Shopping Tip:* Be sure to compare brands of Buffalo wing sauce to avoid added sugars or food starches.

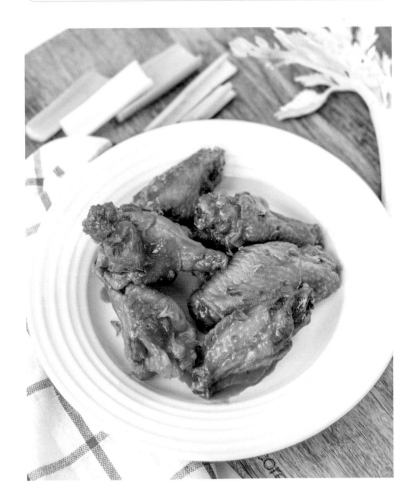

Calories: 387 | Fat: 28.2g | Protein: 24.4g | Carbs: 0.6g | Fiber: 0.1g

# COLD TOSSED PIZZA BOWL

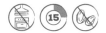

**MAKES** 8 servings
**PREP TIME:** 8 minutes, plus 1 hour to chill

*After sampling about one out of every 100 recipes I make, David looks at me and asks, "How did you do that?" I won't lie, I love that response because it means he likes whatever it is I've made. This is one of those recipes. I created it when we were headed to a get-together and I was empty-handed. A quick tour of the fridge yielded these ingredients, which I cubed, chopped, sliced, diced, and tossed together just before we headed out the door. The guests at the party asked, "Hey, what is this dish? What do you call it?" I confessed that it was something I'd just created and invited the others to name it. Cold Tossed Pizza Bowl is the name that seemed to stick. You can make this a heartier main dish by tossing in some additional meat toppings such as grilled chicken, prosciutto, or browned Italian sausage.*

**8 ounces fresh mozzarella cheese, drained and cubed, or 8 ounces fresh mini mozzarella balls, drained**

**4 ounces pepperoni, chopped**

**⅓ cup chopped roasted red peppers**

**2 tablespoons sun-dried tomatoes in oil, finely diced**

**2 tablespoons finely diced onions**

**1 tablespoon sliced black olives (optional)**

**3 tablespoons avocado oil**

**2 tablespoons balsamic vinegar**

**½ teaspoon dried basil**

**¼ teaspoon Italian seasoning**

**Fresh basil leaves, for garnish (optional)**

Place all the ingredients, except the fresh basil leaves, in a bowl and toss to combine. If time allows, refrigerate for at least 1 hour before serving. Serve in bowls and garnish with fresh basil, if desired. Store leftovers in the refrigerator for up to 5 days.

Calories: 330 | Fat: 24.4g | Protein: 22.9g | Carbs: 4.9g | Fiber: 1g

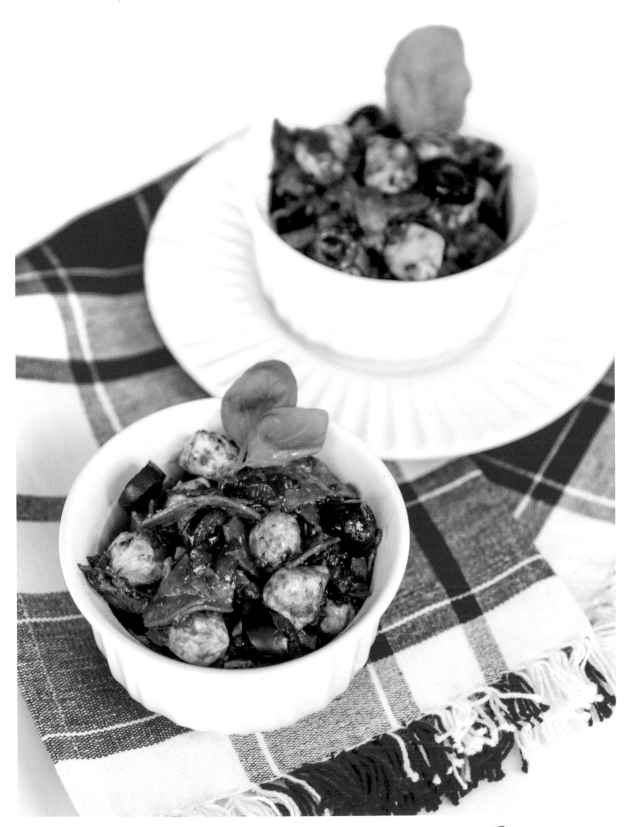

# DECONSTRUCTED CHICKEN CORDON BLEU

**MAKES** 8 servings | **PREP TIME:** 8 minutes, plus 10 minutes to cool (not including time to cook chicken if not purchased precooked) | **COOK TIME:** 40 minutes

*Most people enjoy the subtle flavors of chicken cordon bleu, which includes salty ham, creamy cheese, and breaded chicken, but who has time to make breaded chicken? In this recipe, I have simplified an old favorite by not breading the chicken but including a topping that functions a bit like breading. My family enjoys it, and I suspect yours will, too!*

4 cups shredded cooked chicken

8 slices ham, chopped

8 ounces Swiss or Gruyère cheese, shredded (about 2 cups), divided

2 teaspoons powdered chicken bone broth (optional; see tip, page 62)

1½ cups heavy cream

1 tablespoon Dijon mustard

1 teaspoon Worcestershire sauce

½ cup pork rind dust (see note)

¼ cup shredded Parmesan cheese

2 tablespoons salted butter, softened

Chopped fresh parsley, for garnish (optional)

1. Preheat the oven to 350°F. Grease a 9 by 13-inch baking dish.

2. Place the chicken in an even layer in the prepared baking dish. Top with the ham. Layer 1 cup of the Swiss cheese over the meats.

3. In a small bowl, dissolve the powdered bone broth, if using, into the heavy cream. Stir in the mustard and Worcestershire sauce. Pour the sauce over the chicken, ham, and cheese in the baking dish. Top with the remaining 1 cup of Swiss cheese.

4. In a separate bowl, mix the pork rind dust, Parmesan, and butter with a fork until it resembles coarse sand. Sprinkle the pork rind mixture over the top of the casserole.

5. Bake for 40 to 45 minutes, or until bubbly and lightly browned. Let cool for 10 to 15 minutes before serving. Garnish with fresh parsley, if desired. Store leftovers in the refrigerator for up to 4 days.

*Cook's Note:* Keep pork rind dust on hand at all times! If a bag of pork rinds goes stale and the pork rinds are no longer crisp, toss them in the blender and pulverize them. Store the dust in an airtight container in the pantry until you're ready to use it in recipes like this one.

Calories: 385 | Fat: 32.1g | Protein: 29.1g | Carbs: 3.6g | Fiber: 0.4g

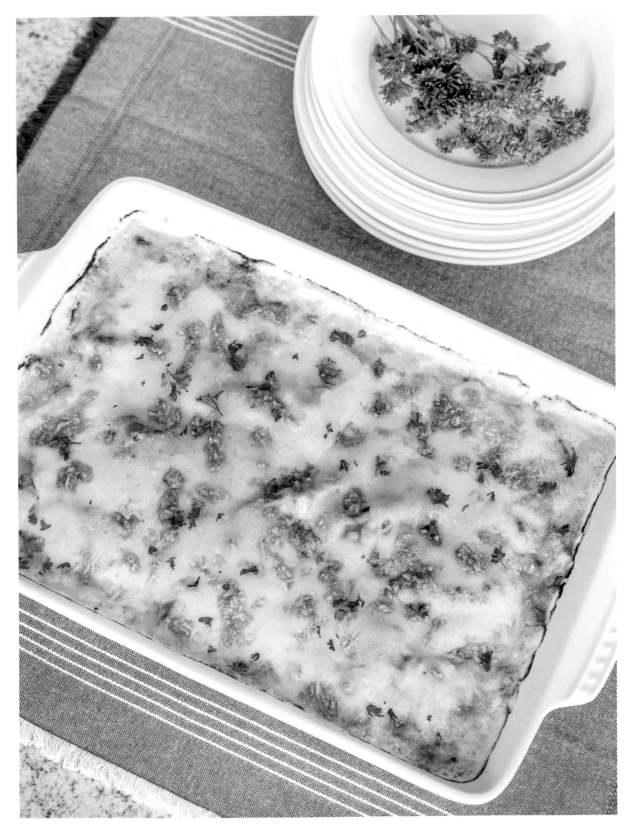

# EASY CHICKEN AND BEEF ENCHILADA BAKE

**MAKES** 6 servings | **PREP TIME:** 10 minutes (not including time to cook chicken if not purchased precooked) | **COOK TIME:** 45 minutes

*Who needs tortillas when we all know that the flavor of enchiladas is in the filling? In this dish, all the ingredients are tossed together and baked into a creamy concoction with as few fattening carbs as possible. You can use only beef or only chicken or replace the beef with chorizo for more flavor if you like. The corn extract, when paired with zucchini, gives this dish a taste and texture that are somewhat similar to those of corn tortillas baked in sauce. Finely dicing the zucchini makes the dish cook more quickly. You can also steam the diced zucchini in the microwave for 2 to 3 minutes before adding it to the recipe to make sure that it cooks thoroughly.*

**1 (10-ounce) can mild red enchilada sauce**

**½ cup sour cream**

**2 ounces cream cheese (¼ cup), softened**

**1 tablespoon taco seasoning**

**1 teaspoon corn extract (optional)**

**3 cups chopped cooked chicken**

**2 cups cooked, crumbled, and drained ground beef**

**1½ cups finely diced zucchini**

**1 (4-ounce) can diced green chilies**

**2 tablespoons seeded and chopped jalapeño peppers**

**2 tablespoons dried minced onion**

**8 ounces Monterey Jack cheese, shredded (about 2 cups), divided**

**4 ounces cheddar cheese, shredded (about 1 cup)**

**¼ cup chopped black olives (optional)**

**Chopped fresh cilantro, for garnish (optional)**

1. Preheat the oven to 350°F. Grease a 9 by 13-inch baking dish.

2. In a large bowl, combine the enchilada sauce, sour cream, cream cheese, taco seasoning, and corn extract, if using. Add the chicken, ground beef, zucchini, chilies, jalapeños, dried minced onion, and 1½ cups of the Monterey Jack cheese. Mix thoroughly and spread in the prepared baking dish. Top with the remaining ½ cup of Monterey Jack cheese, the cheddar cheese, and the black olives, if using.

3. Cover the dish with aluminum foil and bake for 35 to 45 minutes, or until the mixture is bubbling and the zucchini is tender. Remove the foil and bake for an additional 10 to 15 minutes, or until the cheese topping is lightly browned. Serve warm, garnished with fresh cilantro, if desired. Store leftovers in the refrigerator for up to 5 days.

*Crazy Busy Shopping Tip:* Commercial enchilada sauces vary a great deal in terms of ingredients and carb counts. Compare labels and choose the one with the least carbs, preferably without food starches or thickeners. Also, most commercial taco seasonings have added starches such as maltodextrin or have sugar in the mix. One brand that doesn't is Primal Palate Organic Spices.

Calories: 575 | Fat: 34.3g | Protein: 34.1g | Carbs: 5.9g | Fiber: 2.1g

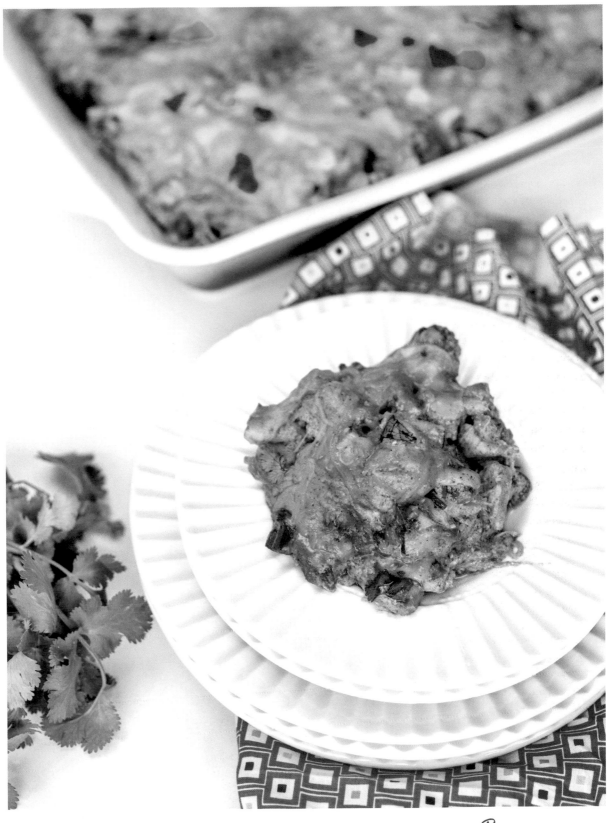

# ONE-PAN CHICKEN ALFREDO WITH SPAGHETTI SQUASH

**MAKES** 6 servings  |  **PREP TIME:** 3 minutes (not including time to cook squash, or to cook chicken if not purchased precooked)  |  **COOK TIME:** 15 minutes

*Like many of the recipes in this book, I created this one while in a hurry. Grace had called to say that she needed to be picked up late from school and then taken to a babysitting job. She would have 15 minutes in the car, and that would be her one chance to eat dinner. I had 20 minutes between getting home from work and leaving to pick her up. I flew into action and made this dish in one large skillet. It was still bubbling when I scooped some into a glass storage container, wrapped the container in a kitchen towel, grabbed a fork, and headed out the door. Grace smiled when she saw it and confided that she had worried what she might have for dinner and when. She handed the empty container to me as I pulled into the driveway of the house where she was babysitting and asked if there might be leftovers for her lunch the next day. I went straight home and stashed some away in the fridge for her before her dad arrived home. We crazy busy people have to stick together!*

¼ cup (½ stick) salted butter

3 cups Microwaved Spaghetti Squash (page 122)

1 teaspoon minced garlic

⅓ cup heavy cream

¼ cup chicken broth

2 ounces cream cheese (¼ cup)

3 cups cubed or shredded cooked chicken

1 teaspoon dried parsley

¼ teaspoon salt

1 cup shredded Parmesan cheese

1.  Melt the butter in a large skillet over high heat. Add the spaghetti squash and garlic and cook, stirring occasionally, until slightly browned.

2.  Reduce the heat to medium and add the heavy cream, broth, and cream cheese. Cook, stirring, until the cream cheese is melted.

3.  Add the chicken, parsley, and salt and stir to combine. Simmer over low heat for 8 to 12 minutes, or until the sauce has thickened. Sprinkle the Parmesan over the dish and serve. Store leftovers in the refrigerator for up to 5 days. Leftovers are best warmed on reduced power in the microwave.

*Crazy Busy Kitchen Tip:* If you microwave the squash and cook the chicken ahead of time, this dish comes together in a snap!

**Calories:** 345 | **Fat:** 22.9g | **Protein:** 23.4g | **Carbs:** 4.3g | **Fiber:** 0.8g

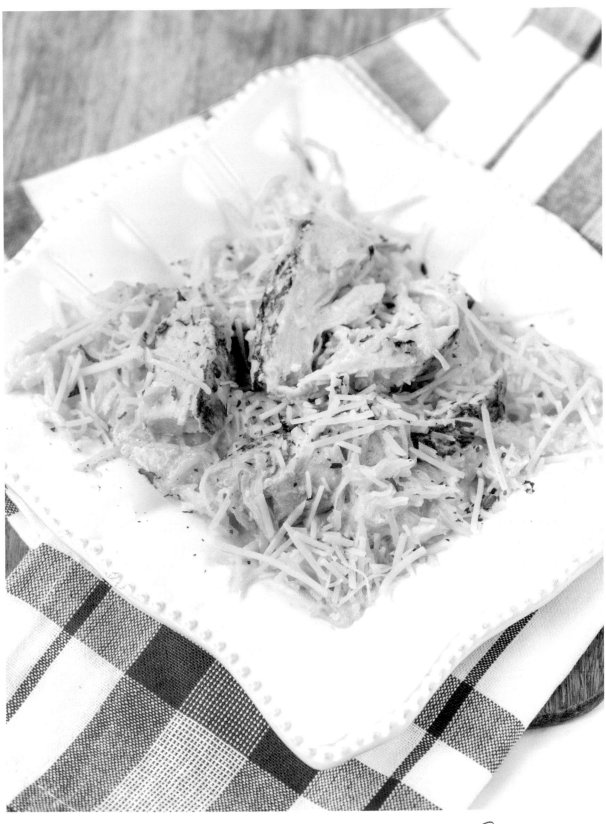

# SHRIMP SALAD-STUFFED AVOCADO BOATS

**MAKES** 2 servings | **PREP TIME:** 6 minutes, plus 20 minutes to chill

*Canned shrimp is a thing? It is! It is an economical and easy thing! Of course, you can use a higher-quality shrimp, finely chopped, but there are advantages to using canned shrimp, including the fact that it's shelf stable and readily available when you need a quick Plan B meal. Except for the cucumbers and tomatoes, this recipe uses staples that I generally keep well stocked. If I happen to find myself without a cucumber or a tomato, I simply leave it out. The cucumbers add a fantastic crunch, but they don't make or break the recipe. In a pinch, you could use 1 tablespoon of finely chopped sun-dried tomatoes instead of fresh tomatoes.*

## DRESSING:

**⅓ cup mayonnaise**

**¼ cup sour cream**

**2 tablespoons lime juice**

**¼ teaspoon minced garlic**

**2 teaspoons dried minced onion**

**1 teaspoon salt**

**Dash of ground black pepper**

**4 (4-ounce) cans tiny shrimp, drained**

**⅓ cup peeled, seeded, and chopped cucumbers**

**⅓ cup chopped tomatoes (optional)**

**1 avocado**

**1.** Make the dressing: In a small mixing bowl, combine the mayonnaise, sour cream, lime juice, garlic, dried minced onion, salt, and pepper.

**2.** In a medium bowl, toss together the shrimp, cucumbers, and tomatoes, if using. Pour the dressing over the shrimp mixture and toss gently to combine. Place in the refrigerator to chill for 20 to 30 minutes before serving.

**3.** To serve, cut the avocado in half and remove the pit. Divide the shrimp salad evenly between the avocado halves. Store leftover salad in the refrigerator for up to 3 days.

Calories: 361 | Fat: 28.4g | Protein: 27.5g | Carbs: 5.4g | Fiber: 2.3g

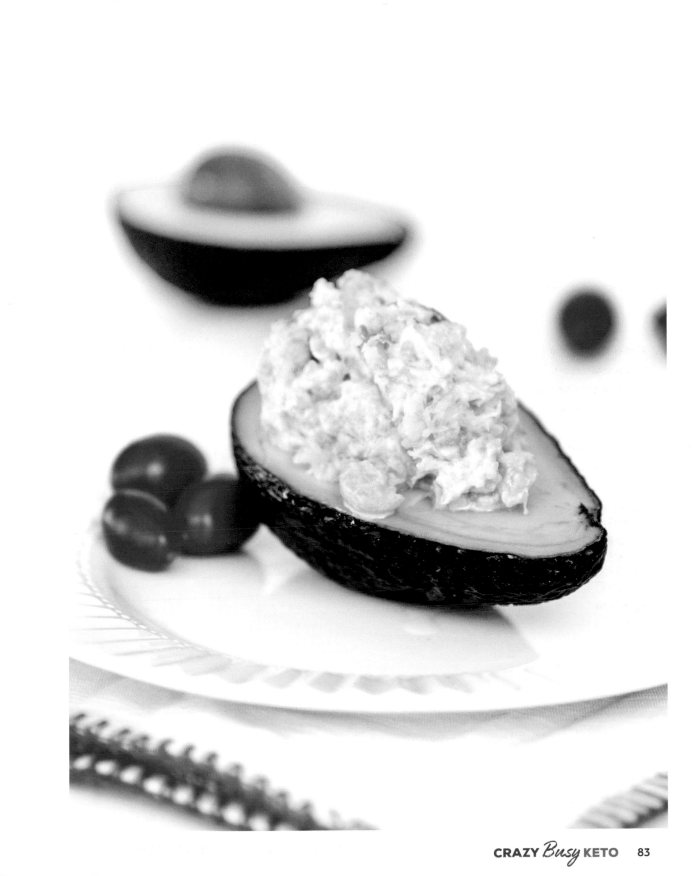

# THAI CHICKEN SLAW WITH PEANUT SAUCE

**MAKES** 4 servings | **PREP TIME:** 5 minutes (not including time to make sauce or cook chicken if not purchased precooked)

*Using bagged coleslaw mix and precooked chicken makes this tasty dish super quick. I often use baked chicken tenderloins; however, rotisserie chicken or even canned chicken works well, too. For the coleslaw mix, I prefer the kind that includes a blend of green cabbage, purple cabbage, and a few shredded carrots. You can make your own, but the bagged coleslaw mix is already washed and chopped and will save you tons of time in the kitchen. Because you will use only about half of the bag of coleslaw mix, you will have half a bag left over to make another batch of this recipe or an easy side of coleslaw. This dish is a great option for lunches. Simply toss the ingredients together and go!*

**8 ounces bagged coleslaw mix (about 3¾ cups)**

**1 cup Thai Peanut Sauce (page 134)**

**1 pound cooked chicken breast tenderloins or chopped or shredded cooked chicken**

**¼ cup sliced green onions (optional)**

**¼ cup salted peanuts (optional)**

1. Put the coleslaw mix and peanut sauce in a large bowl. If using chopped or shredded chicken, add it to the bowl as well. Toss the ingredients until well mixed.

2. Divide the slaw among four plates. If using chicken tenderloins, place them on top of the slaw. Garnish each serving with 1 tablespoon of sliced green onions and 1 tablespoon of peanuts, if desired. Store leftovers in the refrigerator for up to 2 days.

*Cook's Note:* This dish is also fantastic warm. If you have time, you can stir-fry the coleslaw mix in 1 to 2 tablespoons of ghee, bacon fat, or avocado oil. Add the chicken to the skillet to warm it through, remove the pan from the heat, and add the sauce. Toss well and serve.

*Crazy Busy Kitchen Tip:* Make a batch of Thai Peanut Sauce on Sunday evening and refrigerate it until you are ready to use it. It will keep for up to 1 week, and it gets even better over time. It's great with any type of salad or protein such as shrimp or pork.

Calories: 215 | Fat: 4.9g | Protein: 33.6g | Carbs: 2.9g | Fiber: 1.8g

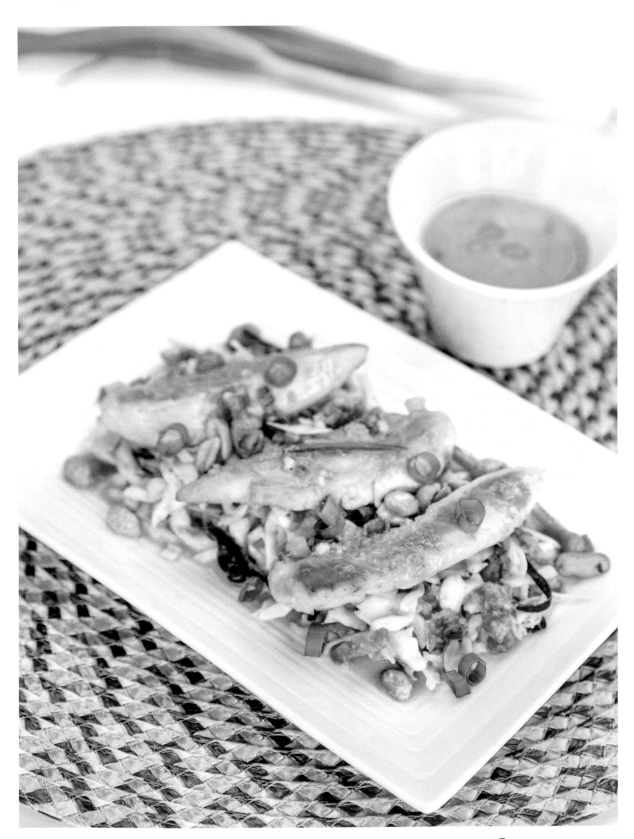

# FRIED SALMON PATTIES

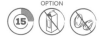

**MAKES** 6 servings
**PREP TIME:** 5 minutes | **COOK TIME:** 8 minutes

*My grandmother used to make the best salmon patties! She crushed up saltines to add to the salmon mixture. As a child of the Great Depression, I'm sure this helped to stretch her grocery budget. Instead of crackers or breadcrumbs, my recipe uses finely crushed pork rinds and Parmesan cheese. Not only do these ingredients serve as binders, but they also give the salmon patties a wonderful flavor.*

**PATTIES:**

1 (14.75-ounce) can salmon, drained

⅓ cup mayonnaise, plus extra for serving if desired

⅓ cup pork rind dust

¼ cup shredded Parmesan cheese (omit for dairy-free)

2 large eggs, beaten

2 teaspoons dried minced onion

2 teaspoons dried parsley

2 teaspoons lemon juice

1 teaspoon Worcestershire sauce

2 tablespoons bacon fat, ghee, or avocado oil, for frying

Chopped fresh parsley, for garnish (optional)

Lemon wedges, for serving (optional)

1. Place all the ingredients for the patties in a large mixing bowl and mix until thoroughly combined. Shape into patties 2 to 2½ inches in diameter and about ¼ inch thick. You should get about 12 patties.

2. Heat the fat in a large skillet over medium heat. Place the patties in the hot fat, leaving at least ½ inch between them. Reduce the heat to medium-low and fry the patties for 4 to 6 minutes on each side, or until lightly browned.

3. Serve warm with a dollop of mayonnaise and/or lemon wedges and garnish with parsley, if desired. Store leftovers in the refrigerator for up to 4 days.

**Calories:** 418 | **Fat:** 38.5g | **Protein:** 20.4g | **Carbs:** 0.6g | **Fiber:** 0g

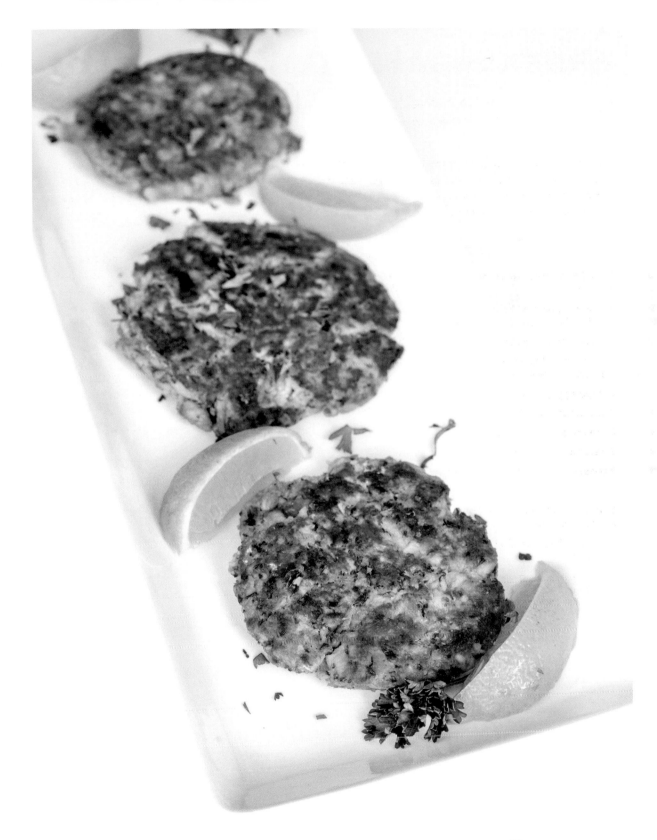

# GREEK MEATBALLS

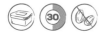

**MAKES** 8 servings  |  **PREP TIME:** 8 minutes (not including time to cook spinach)
**COOK TIME:** 15 minutes

*Lamb has always seemed like an exotic meat to me because it's something I didn't grow up eating. Maybe that's why I enjoy it so much as an adult. In this recipe, I like to combine lamb and beef, but you could use all lamb or all beef if you prefer. The mint is subtle but offers an authentic Greek flavor, especially when combined with the spinach and feta. We enjoy these served with the Tzatziki Sauce on page 132. To save time, you can form the meat mixture into mini meatloaves instead of meatballs; see the variation below.*

**1 pound ground beef**

**1 pound ground lamb**

**1 (10-ounce) package frozen spinach, cooked and drained well**

**1½ tablespoons chopped fresh mint, or 2 teaspoons dried mint**

**1 tablespoon dried minced onion**

**2 teaspoons minced garlic**

**½ teaspoon salt**

**4 ounces feta cheese, crumbled (about 1 cup)**

**1.**  Preheat the oven to 375°F. Line a large rimmed baking sheet with parchment paper.

**2.**  Place all the ingredients in a large mixing bowl and use your hands to thoroughly combine. Shape the mixture into 1½-inch balls and place on the lined baking sheet, spacing them about ½ inch apart. You should get about 40 meatballs.

**3.**  Bake for 15 to 20 minutes, or until cooked through. Serve warm. Store leftovers in the refrigerator for up to 4 days.

*Crazy Busy Kitchen Tip:* These meatballs freeze well and can be portioned into freezer bags. For brown-bag lunches, they can be taken straight from the freezer in the morning and will be thawed and ready to eat by lunchtime. Make an extra batch and freeze half for future meals.

**Variation: Greek Mini Meatloaves.** After mixing all the ingredients together, press the mixture evenly into four 5¾ by 3-inch mini meatloaf pans. Bake for 20 to 25 minutes, or until the juices run clear when cut.

Calories: 348 | Fat: 15.3g | Protein: 30.1g | Carbs: 2.6g | Fiber: 1.1g

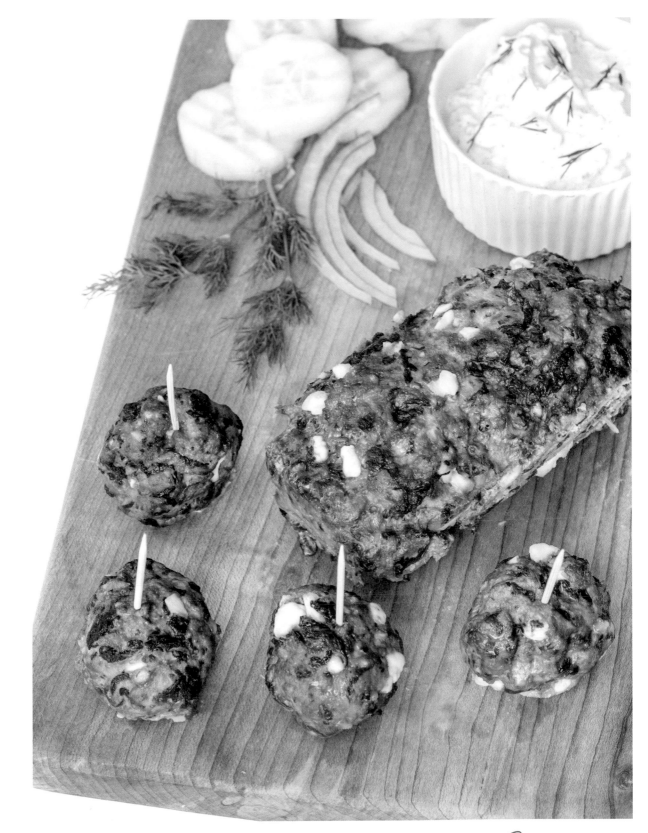

# QUICK CHICKEN CHOWDER

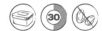 **MAKES** 6 servings | **PREP TIME:** 4 minutes (not including time to cook bacon or chicken if not purchased precooked) | **COOK TIME:** 25 minutes

*Soup's on and dinner's done! This chowder is truly fast when you use dried minced onion, frozen cauliflower, and precooked bacon and chicken. Once you toss everything together, just let it simmer while you slip out of your work clothes and call the family to the table. While the corn extract is optional, it adds a more authentic corn flavor that is typically associated with corn chowder.*

¼ cup (½ stick) salted butter

½ medium onion, chopped, or
2 tablespoons dried minced onion

2 cups chopped cauliflower stems
and florets

2 cups chicken broth

½ cup chopped cooked bacon

1 cup heavy cream

3 ounces cream cheese

1 tablespoon dried parsley

2 teaspoons garlic powder

¼ teaspoon salt

1½ pounds chopped cooked
chicken

2 teaspoons corn extract
(optional)

1. Melt the butter in a medium saucepan over medium heat. Sauté the chopped onion in the butter until it just begins to brown. (If using dried minced onion, wait to add it until the cream is added.)

2. Stir in the cauliflower and broth. Bring to a simmer, then add the bacon, heavy cream, cream cheese, parsley, garlic powder, and salt. Stir until the cream cheese is melted.

3. Reduce the heat to low and simmer for 15 to 18 minutes, or until the cauliflower is tender and the broth has thickened. Stir in the chicken and corn extract, if using, and continue heating until the chicken is warmed. Serve hot. Store leftovers in the refrigerator for up to 5 days.

*Crazy Busy Kitchen Tip: Make a double batch of chowder and freeze it in 1½-cup portions for future meals.*

**Calories:** 420 | **Fat:** 26.6g | **Protein:** 36.3g | **Carbs:** 3.1g | **Fiber:** 1.1g

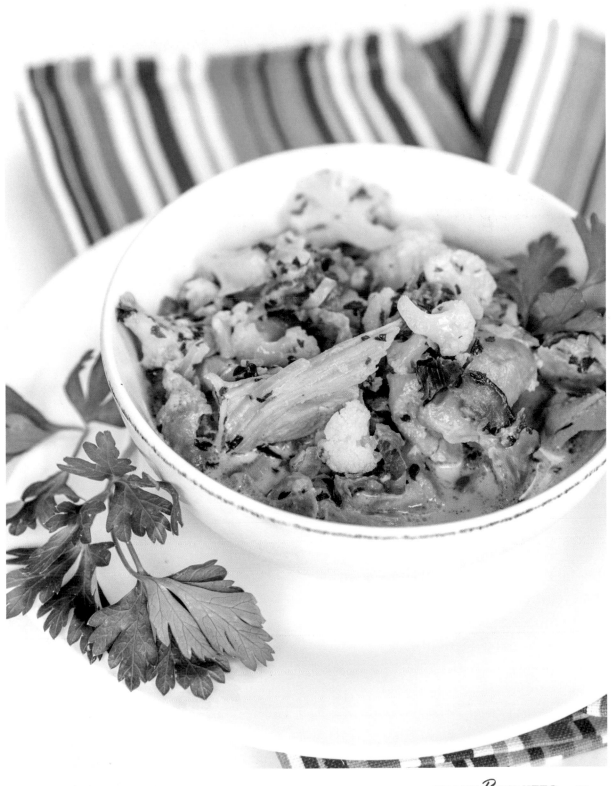

# EASY EGG AND BACON SALAD

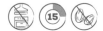

**MAKES** 2 servings  |  **PREP TIME:** 5 minutes (not including time to cook eggs or bacon if not purchased precooked)

*My mother made a simple egg salad with mayo, mustard, salt, and pepper. This recipe is not much more complex, except that I like to add cream cheese and bacon. You can consider this a Plan B recipe, as you're likely to have most of the ingredients on hand. You can also easily purchase these ingredients while traveling and make this simple egg salad on the go using only a bowl and a plastic knife and fork.*

**⅓ cup mayonnaise**

**2 ounces cream cheese (¼ cup), softened**

**1½ teaspoons prepared yellow mustard**

**¼ teaspoon salt**

**¼ teaspoon ground black pepper**

**6 hard-boiled eggs, peeled and finely chopped**

**2 tablespoons cooked bacon pieces**

**1 green onion (green part only), thinly sliced (optional)**

In a mixing bowl, use a fork to mix the mayonnaise, cream cheese, mustard, salt, and pepper until smooth. Add the eggs, bacon, and green onion, if using, and stir until well combined.

*Crazy Busy Kitchen Tip:* Save time by using packaged hard-boiled eggs from the refrigerated section of the grocery store. (They're usually found near the raw eggs.) The pre-boiled eggs are already shelled, which leaves you more time to enjoy your meal!

**Calories:** 357 | **Fat:** 31.5g | **Protein:** 22.9g | **Carbs:** 1.9g | **Fiber:** 0.5g

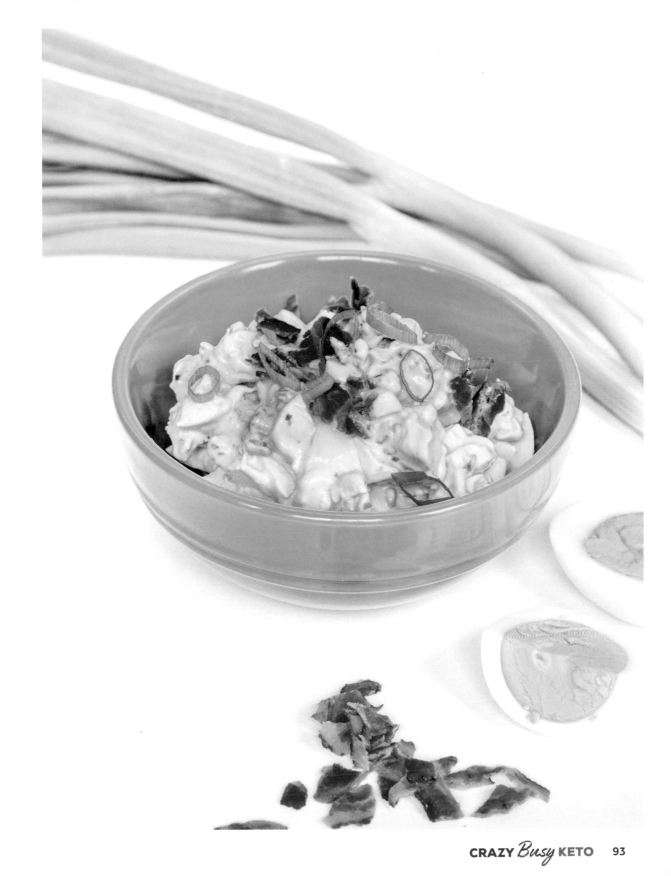

# PAN-SEARED STEAK

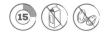

**MAKES** 2 servings | **PREP TIME:** 1 minute
**COOK TIME:** 6 to 10 minutes, depending on desired doneness

*This is my family's favorite quick meal. Although I never thought of steak as fast, once I started paying attention, I realized that a great steak is one of the quickest and easiest meals anyone can make. The key is knowing how to cook it. Because I have a gas cooktop, I like to sear steaks in a cast-iron skillet. I turn the heat up as high as it will go to preheat the skillet really well before putting the steak in the pan. Be sure to turn on the ventilation for the cooktop, too. If the steak doesn't sizzle when it hits the pan, then the skillet isn't hot enough. With regard to serving size, keep in mind that 3 to 4 ounces of meat is one standard serving. You can always eat a larger portion if you prefer. I often serve steak with a pat of butter on top for extra fat and flavor.*

**1 (10-ounce) rib-eye steak (½ inch thick)**

**⅛ teaspoon garlic powder**

**Dash of salt**

**Dash of ground black pepper**

**1 tablespoon bacon fat or avocado oil**

1. Season the steak on both sides with the garlic powder, salt, and pepper and set aside.

2. Heat the fat in a 9-inch cast-iron skillet over high heat just until it begins to smoke. Use a pair of tongs to carefully place the steak in the skillet. Set a timer and cook the steak to your desired doneness:

   3 minutes on each side for rare (red inside)

   4 minutes on each side for medium (dark pink in the center)

   5 minutes on each side for well-done (no pink in the center)

3. After searing the steak on the second side, remove from the skillet and serve warm.

*Cook's Note:* Leftover steak can be used in omelets, frittatas, or Salad Bar Stir-Fry (page 96).

Calories: 303 | Fat: 18g | Protein: 33.4g | Carbs: 0.2g | Fiber: 0g

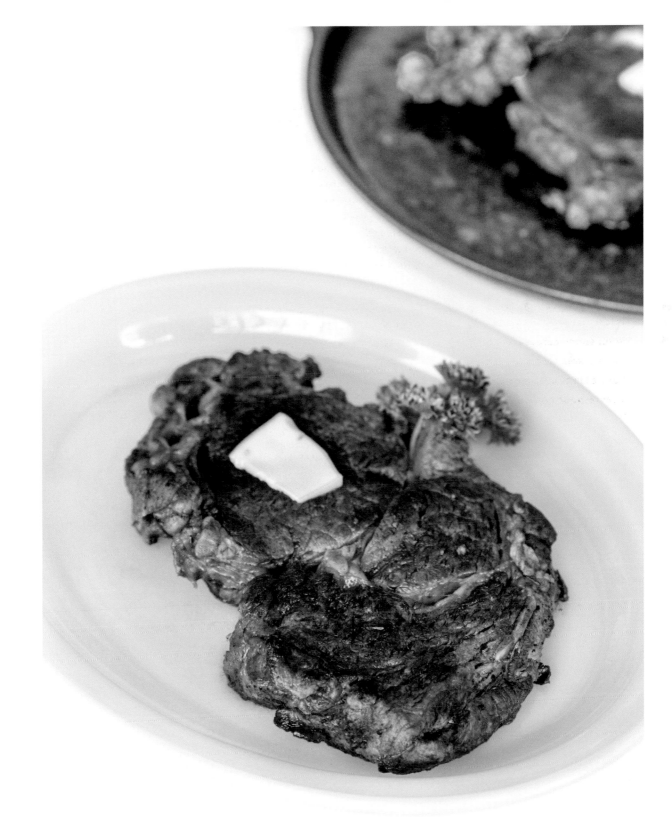

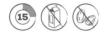

# SALAD BAR STIR-FRY

**MAKES** 2 servings
**PREP TIME:** 2 minutes | **COOK TIME:** 11 minutes

*This recipe is the ultimate cheap and lazy idea, and I love that it saves room in my fridge and keeps me from buying a lot of unnecessary vegetables that eventually would go bad and be thrown away. With this simple stir-fry, I can enjoy a variety of fresh vegetables and know that nothing will go to waste. In fact, when I made this recipe for photos, I spent just $1.84 on the vegetables! The secret? Buy them from the grocery store salad bar. You can grab a lot of different veggies that are already cleaned and chopped. If I had purchased a head of broccoli, a head of cauliflower, a container of mushrooms, a head of cabbage, an onion, a bunch of celery, and a bag of spinach, I easily would have spent $12 or more, and I might have thrown most of the leftovers away because I was too busy to cook them all. My Salad Bar Stir-Fry uses only small amounts of veggies and can easily be tweaked depending on which fresh veggies you prefer to grab from the salad bar.*

2 tablespoons bacon fat, ghee, or avocado oil

2 ounces cauliflower florets (about ¾ cup), chopped

2 ounces broccoli florets (about ½ cup), chopped

1 ounce sliced mushrooms (about ⅓ cup)

1 ounce chopped bell peppers (any color) (about ⅓ cup)

1 ounce chopped purple cabbage (about ¼ cup)

2 tablespoons chopped celery

2 tablespoons chopped red onions

1 teaspoon minced garlic, or ½ teaspoon garlic powder

8 ounces chopped cooked chicken

⅓ cup spinach leaves

4 grape tomatoes, halved

¼ teaspoon salt

Dash of ground black pepper

2 tablespoons coconut aminos or soy sauce

1. Heat the fat in a large skillet over medium-high heat. Add the cauliflower, broccoli, mushrooms, bell peppers, cabbage, celery, red onions, and garlic and stir-fry until crisp-tender, 8 to 10 minutes.

2. Add the chicken, spinach, and tomatoes to the skillet and stir-fry until the spinach is just wilted and the chicken is warmed, 3 to 5 minutes.

3. Season with the salt and pepper and serve immediately. Drizzle the coconut aminos over the skillet or over each plate just before serving.

Calories: 332 | Fat: 17.8g | Protein: 24.5g | Carbs: 5.5g | Fiber: 2.4g

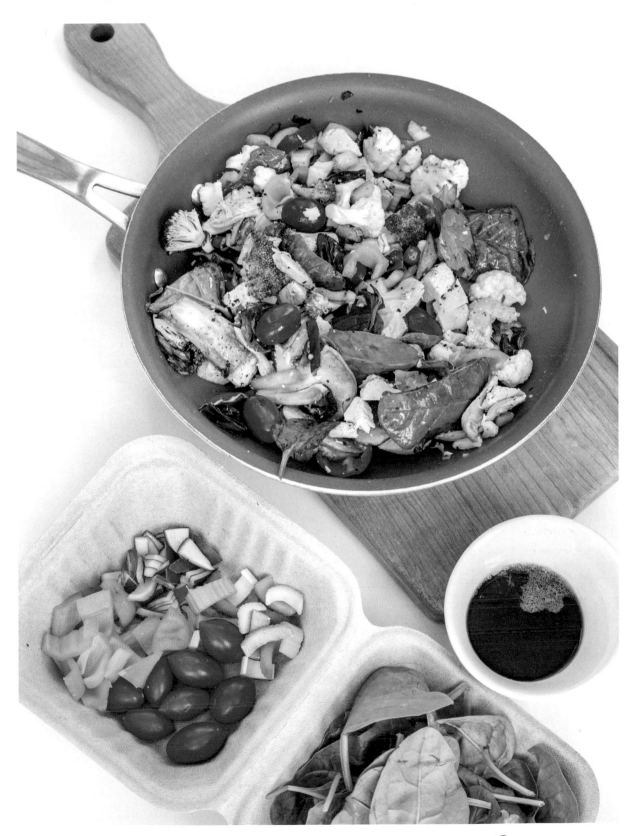

# LAZY SLOW COOKER BEEF STEW

**MAKES** 8 servings
**PREP TIME:** 5 minutes | **COOK TIME:** 6 hours

*My little carbivore Jonathan sometimes asks for beef stew. I don't mind honoring his request since it's as simple as putting everything into a slow cooker, setting it, and then dishing out dinner eight hours later, but I do avoid adding the starchy potatoes and carrots that are traditionally included. So far, he hasn't noticed or complained! The meat creates its own rich broth that can be simmered down and thickened just before serving. You can make cauli rice or cauli mash as a quick side. To speed things up, use frozen riced cauliflower or frozen florets.*

3 pounds beef stew meat

1 pound radishes, trimmed (large ones halved)

8 ounces mushrooms, sliced

½ onion, sliced

1 medium stalk celery, chopped (about ⅓ cup)

½ cup (1 stick) salted butter, cut into pieces

2 teaspoons Worcestershire sauce

3 bay leaves (optional)

1 teaspoon garlic powder

1 teaspoon onion powder

1 teaspoon salt

⅛ teaspoon ground black pepper

1. Place the meat in a 4-quart or larger slow cooker. Cover with the remaining ingredients. Cook on low for 6 to 8 hours, or until the beef is fork-tender. Remove the bay leaves, if used, before serving.

2. If desired, remove the meat and veggies to a bowl and pour the cooking liquid into a medium saucepan. Simmer over medium heat for 6 to 10 minutes, or until the broth has thickened, then pour the thickened broth over the meat and veggies. Serve warm. Store leftovers in the refrigerator for up to 4 days.

Calories: 349 | Fat: 22.3g | Protein: 28.2g | Carbs: 4.3g | Fiber: 1.4g

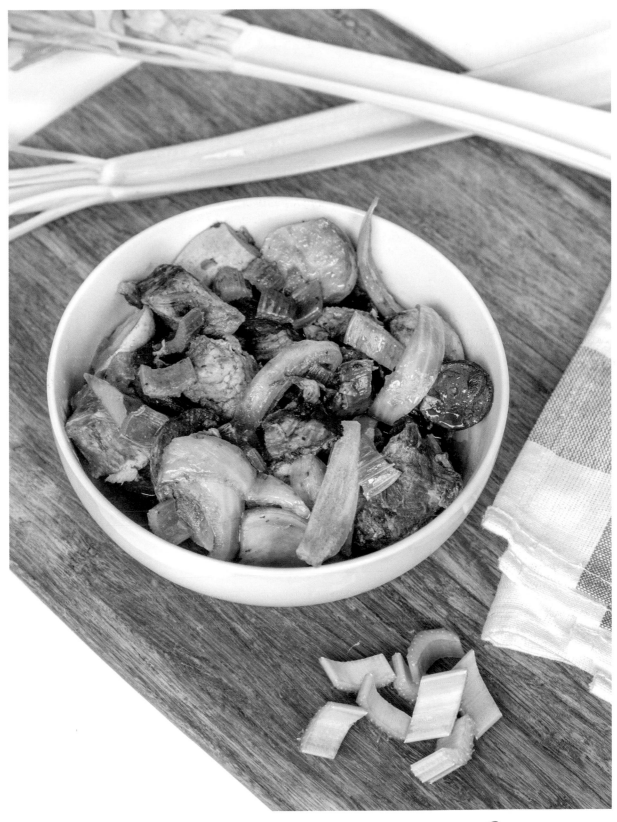

# SPICY POPPIN' SHRIMP

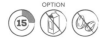

**MAKES** 4 servings
**PREP TIME:** 8 minutes  |  **COOK TIME:** 4 minutes

*The restaurant version of this recipe uses small shrimp that are breaded and fried, but after trying it with sautéed shrimp, I realized that the magic really is in the sauce and not in the breading. The sauce is simple and uses common ingredients; you can use more or less Sriracha depending on how spicy you want it to be. A sprinkling of pork rind dust at the end gives the dish just a hint of the traditional breading texture but can easily be omitted. You can also use chopped cooked chicken or another type of seafood in place of the shrimp.*

**SAUCE:**

½ cup mayonnaise

¼ cup chili garlic sauce

1½ teaspoons lemon juice

1 teaspoon Sriracha sauce

3 drops liquid sweetener

2 pounds raw medium shrimp, peeled and deveined

2 tablespoons salted butter or refined coconut oil

**FOR SERVING:**

2 cups shredded iceberg lettuce

¼ cup pork rind dust (optional)

1 green onion, sliced (optional)

1.  Make the sauce: In a large bowl, whisk together the mayonnaise, chili garlic sauce, lemon juice, Sriracha, and sweetener. Set aside.

2.  Pat the shrimp dry. Melt the butter in a large skillet over medium-high heat. Sauté the shrimp in the butter until it just turns pink and is cooked through, 4 to 6 minutes. Remove the shrimp from the skillet with a slotted spoon and place in the bowl with the sauce. Toss to coat.

3.  To serve, divide the lettuce among four plates. Serve the shrimp over the top of the lettuce. If desired, sprinkle the pork rind dust and sliced green onion over the shrimp just before serving. Store leftovers in the refrigerator (keeping the sauced shrimp separate from the lettuce) for up to 3 days.

*Crazy Busy Shopping Tip:* Remember to look for chili garlic sauce, not sweet chili sauce. The brand I use is Huy Fong Foods.

*Crazy Busy Kitchen Tip:* Make the sauce up to 1 week in advance so that you can make a quick meal without dirtying a second bowl.

Calories: 365 | Fat: 26.4g | Protein: 25.1g | Carbs: 4.9g | Fiber: 0.7g

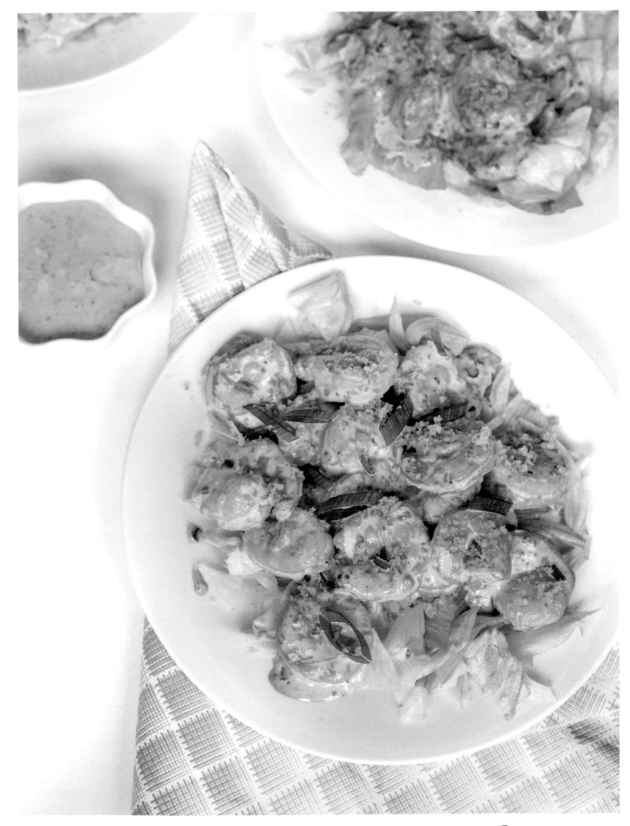

# EGG DROP SOUP

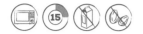

**MAKES** 1 serving
**PREP TIME:** 3 minutes  |  **COOK TIME:** 8 minutes

*We call this comfort food at my house because it's perfect for those times when your tummy feels a little off. It's also great when you need some protein that's fast, inexpensive, and comes with minimal cleanup. While I've provided directions for making the soup on the stovetop, you can also cook it in the microwave at full power, which makes it a good option when you don't have a full kitchen but you do have a microwave.*

**2 cups chicken broth**

**1 tablespoon sliced green onions, or ¼ teaspoon dried minced onion**

**⅛ teaspoon garlic powder**

**2 large eggs, beaten**

**¼ teaspoon toasted sesame oil**

**¼ teaspoon coconut aminos (optional)**

**Dash of salt**

**Dash of ground black pepper**

Bring the broth to a boil in a medium saucepan over medium-high heat. Add the onions and garlic powder. Very slowly pour in the beaten eggs, stirring continuously. When the eggs are cooked, 2 to 3 minutes, pour the soup into a serving bowl. Top with the sesame oil, coconut aminos (if using), salt, and pepper. Serve immediately.

*Crazy Busy Shopping Tip:* If using prepared broth rather than homemade, look for brands with few ingredients. Avoid potato starch, maltodextrin, sugar, corn syrup, and other added carbs.

Calories: 233 | Fat: 13.8g | Protein: 16.4g | Carbs: 1.5g | Fiber: 0.2g

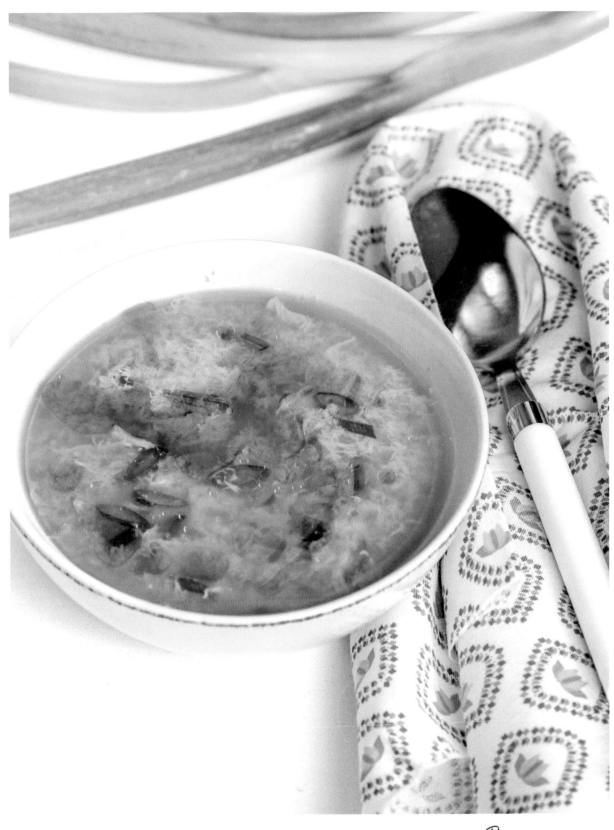

# CHAPTER 3

# CRAZY *Busy* SIDES & SAUCES

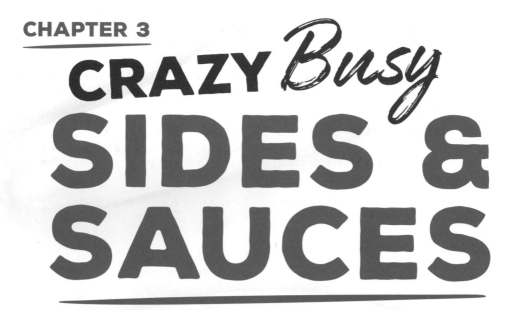

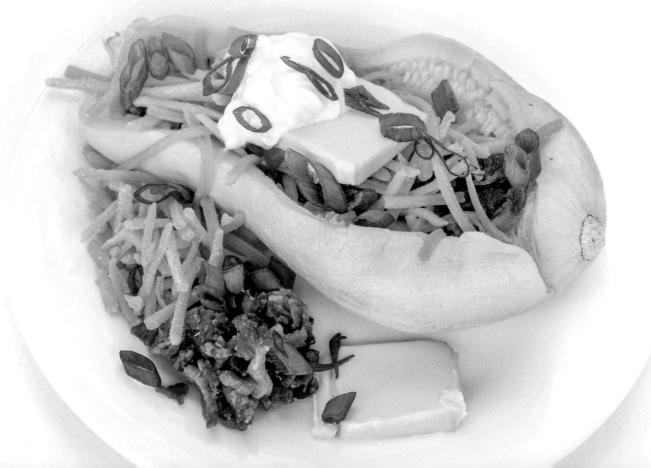

Side dishes often highlight vegetables, but they should also be a primary vehicle for fat, which equals flavor. Because most of the recipes in the Main Dishes chapter are complete meals, I've minimized the number of sides included in this book, choosing only those that are truly fast or can be transformed into a filling main dish just by adding a source of protein. For example, the Mexican Fiesta Cauli Rice becomes a hearty meal when you add cooked chicken or beef, just like the One-Bowl Creamed Spinach and Artichokes, which also can be prepared in a microwave if your access to a kitchen is limited.

I've taken great care to include sides that require little more than a knife, a mixing bowl, utensils, and a means to measure ingredients. Not only do these recipes require minimal cleanup, but many of them can be put together while traveling or camping, with several being perfect for dorm life.

Just because I've chosen simple recipes with few ingredients doesn't mean that you won't enjoy these sides. Because of the added fat and extraordinary flavor, many of them will easily steal the show.

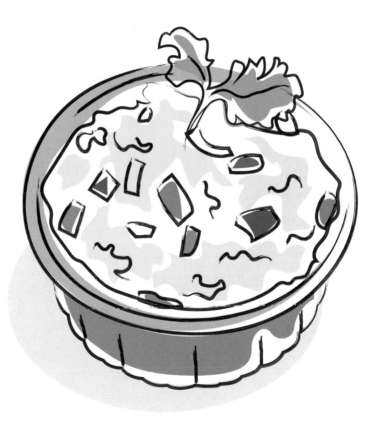

# SUPER *Speedy* SIDES

When there's no time for recipes, sides can be really simple. Look to your pantry or freezer stash for ideas (see the shopping lists on pages 12 to 16). Steam, fry, or roast for simplicity. Add fats—butter for flavor, avocado oil or ghee for frying, and bacon fat or refined coconut oil for roasting. Here are a few ideas from my Crazy Busy Kitchen.

## GREEN BEANS WITH HAM OR BACON

If using canned green beans, drain half of the liquid before putting the remaining contents in a saucepan. Add 1 ounce of chopped country ham or three strips of crumbled precooked bacon. Let simmer, covered, for 10 minutes. Remove the lid and simmer for an additional 3 to 5 minutes, or until most of the moisture has evaporated. Add 2 tablespoons of salted butter and serve immediately.

If using frozen green beans, place the green beans in a saucepan along with ½ cup of water. Add ham or bacon as directed above, and simmer, covered, for 15 to 20 minutes, or until the green beans are tender. Finish cooking and serve as directed above.

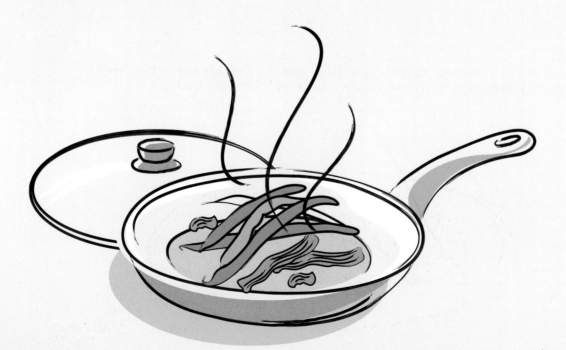

## RICED CAULIFLOWER

Pan-fry frozen riced cauliflower in 2 tablespoons of salted butter or ghee until tender. Season with salt to taste.

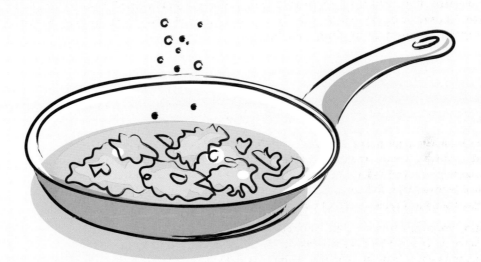

## LOADED BROCCOLI

Steam frozen broccoli until tender. Drain well and top with salted butter. Serve with shredded cheese, chopped cooked bacon, and a dollop of sour cream.

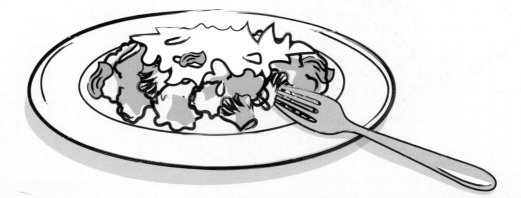

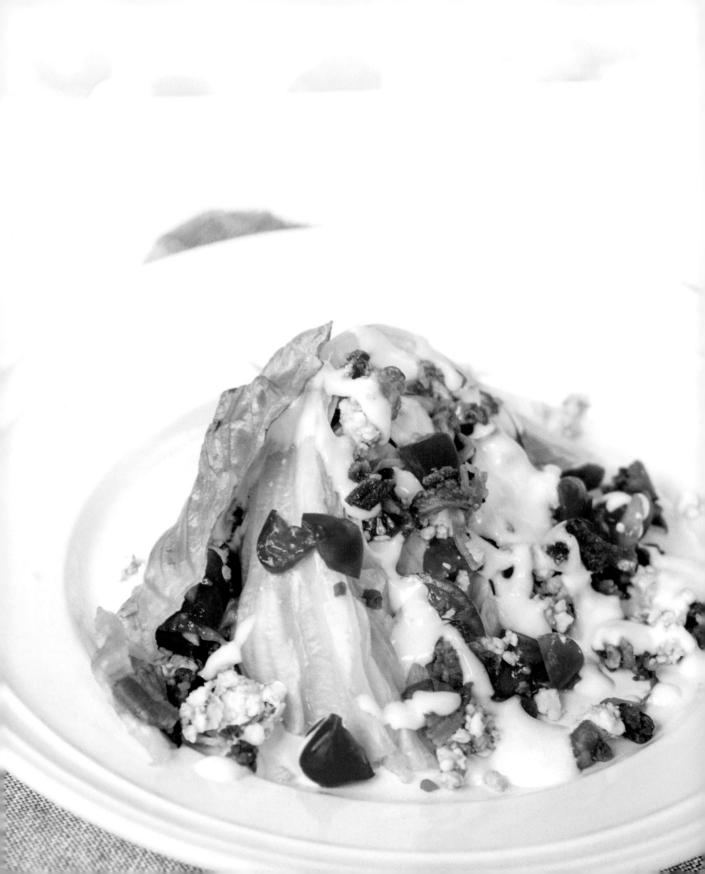

# Recipes

# ONE-BOWL CREAMED SPINACH AND ARTICHOKES

**MAKES** 6 servings
**PREP TIME:** 2 minutes | **COOK TIME:** 3 minutes, plus time to cook frozen spinach

*For this recipe, I adapted a popular dish to be made in a microwave. As long as your microwave is large enough to hold a medium-sized bowl, you can make this dish anywhere, including a hotel room or office kitchen, provided that you have a can opener, a spoon or rubber spatula, and all of the simple ingredients on hand. For a complete meal with plenty of protein, add a small can of cooked chicken or serve this as a side with beef, chicken, or fish. Look for artichoke hearts packed in water rather than in oil. I also tend to purchase frozen spinach that comes in plastic pouches. I cook the spinach in the microwave while I assemble the other ingredients, then pierce the plastic with a fork and drain the liquid into the sink. The spinach doesn't need to be squeezed dry, just drained of most of the water in the package.*

**1 (10-ounce) package frozen spinach, cooked and drained**

**1 (8-ounce) package cream cheese**

**1 (14-ounce) can quartered artichoke hearts, drained and chopped**

**⅓ cup mayonnaise**

**1 teaspoon onion powder**

**½ teaspoon garlic powder**

**Dash of ground black pepper**

**⅛ teaspoon salt**

**6 ounces shredded Parmesan cheese (about 1½ cups)**

1. Place the cooked spinach, cream cheese, and artichoke hearts in a medium microwave-safe bowl and heat at 70% power for 1 minute. Stir until the cream cheese is smooth and all the ingredients are well mixed. Heat in additional 30-second increments on reduced power as needed. When creamy, stir in the mayonnaise, spices, and salt until combined. Add the Parmesan cheese and mix well.

2. Return the bowl to the microwave and cook on 70% power for up to 1 minute, or until creamy and just bubbly. (Alternatively, you can heat only the portion you wish to eat and refrigerate the rest for another meal.) Stir well before serving. Store leftovers in the refrigerator for up to 5 days.

> *Cook's Notes:* My microwave is 1250 watts. If yours has a lower wattage, you may need to increase the cook time a bit.
>
> If you add an 8-ounce can of cooked chicken to make this a full meal, increase the mayonnaise to ½ cup. Be sure to drain the chicken before adding it to the bowl with the creamed spinach and artichokes.
>
> If you have time, the spinach mixture can be spread in an 8-inch square baking dish and baked at 350°F for 15 to 20 minutes, or until lightly browned and bubbly.
>
> This recipe makes a fairly large batch. If you won't be consuming all of it right away, complete Step 1, then heat only the portion you plan to serve immediately. Store in single-serving portions for ease.

Calories: 302 | Fat: 23.8g | Protein: 18.2g | Carbs: 4.7g | Fiber: 2.9g

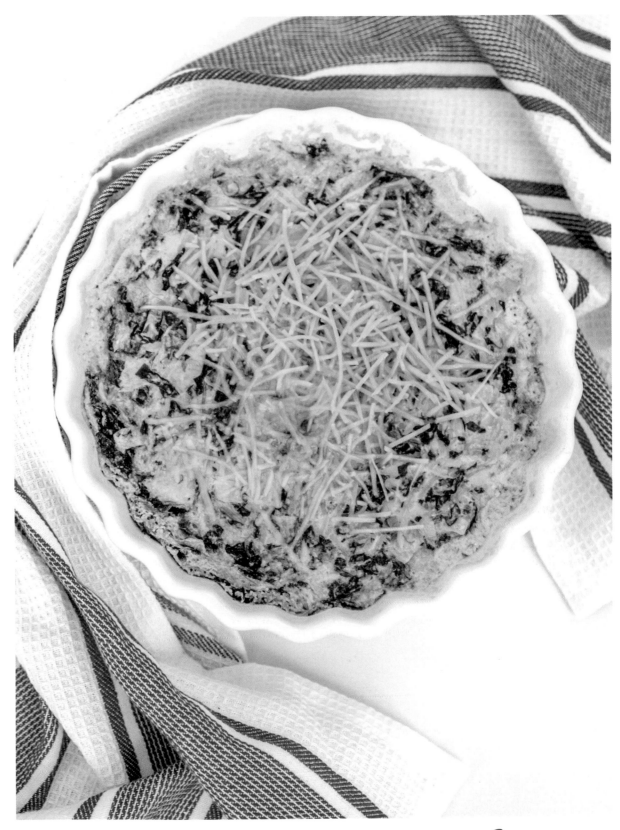

# SIMPLE WEDGE SALAD

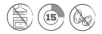

**MAKES** 4 servings  |  **PREP TIME:** 4 minutes (not including time to cook bacon or eggs if not purchased precooked)

*Yes, this salad is incredibly simple and fast, and I promise that if you use a head of super fresh iceberg lettuce, you'll wonder why you don't eat it more often! Every time I make this recipe, I wonder why it tastes so much better than a salad made with shredded lettuce. My only guess is that it's related to the crisp, fresh taste of the lettuce. If you're making only one serving, I suggest cutting a wedge and leaving the rest of the head of lettuce intact; it will stay fresher that way. You might get six to eight wedges depending on the size of the head of lettuce and your preferred serving size. You can add canned tuna, rotisserie chicken, Pan-Seared Steak (page 94), or nearly any other protein you like. Lastly, if you aren't a fan of blue cheese, you can swap out the blue cheese crumbles for shredded cheddar and use ranch dressing instead. My family prefers it this way.*

**1 small head iceberg lettuce**

**1 cup crumbled cooked bacon**

**1 medium tomato, chopped, or 8 to 10 grape tomatoes, or a combination**

**4 ounces blue cheese, crumbled (about 1 cup)**

**2 hard-boiled eggs, peeled and sliced (optional)**

**1 cup blue cheese dressing**

1. Rinse the head of lettuce in cold water and drain. Pat the outside dry with a clean kitchen towel. Use a knife to cut the head in half, then cut each half in two to create four wedges.

2. Place each wedge on a plate with a cut side down. Top each wedge with ¼ cup of the bacon crumbles, one-quarter of the chopped tomato, 1 ounce of the blue cheese crumbles, and one-quarter of the egg slices, if using. Drizzle ¼ cup of dressing over the top of each salad and serve immediately. Uncut lettuce wedges and toppings can be refrigerated separately for up to 3 days and then combined for a quick meal or a lunch on the go.

*Crazy Busy Kitchen Tip:* Use store-bought precooked bacon or bacon pieces, purchase blue cheese already crumbled, buy eggs that are already hard-boiled, and use prepared blue cheese dressing.

*Crazy Busy Travel Tip:* Take packaged ingredients (precut) on the road with you for an easy hotel, office, or RV camping meal—anywhere you have access to a cooler or refrigeration.

**Calories:** 285 | **Fat:** 24.1g | **Protein:** 13.8g | **Carbs:** 4.2g | **Fiber:** 1.2g

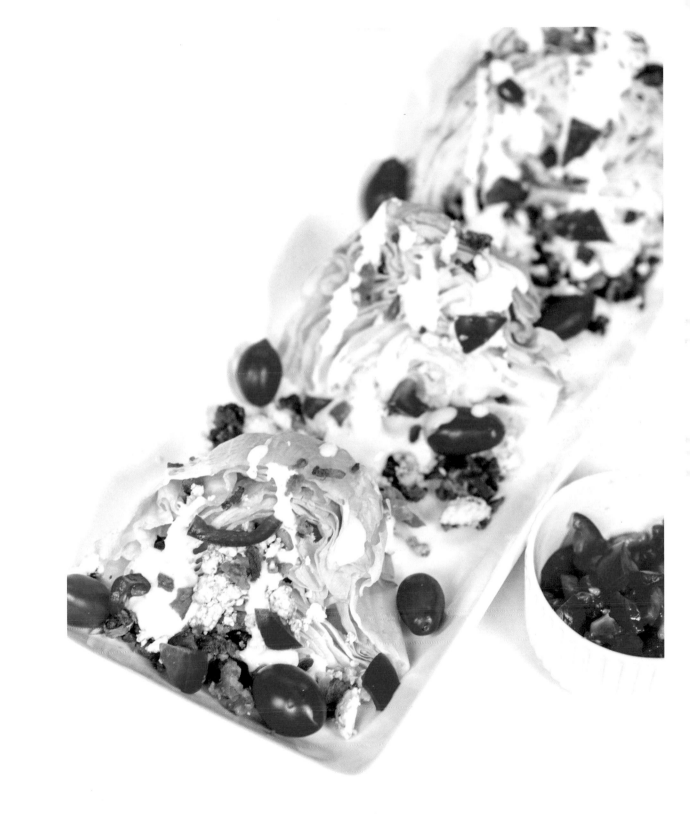

# PAN-FRIED CAULIFLOWER WITH PESTO

**MAKES** 8 servings (about ½ cup per serving)
**PREP TIME:** 6 minutes | **COOK TIME:** 8 minutes

*To make this recipe even faster, start with frozen cauliflower florets. The key to outstanding flavor is to pan-fry the cauliflower over high heat just until it's nicely browned and tender; if overcooked, the cauliflower will become mushy.*

2 tablespoons bacon fat, avocado oil, or refined coconut oil

4 cups chopped cauliflower florets

½ cup prepared pesto sauce

¼ teaspoon red pepper flakes (optional)

¼ cup shredded Parmesan cheese (optional)

1. Heat the bacon fat in a large skillet over high heat. Add the cauliflower and pan-fry in the bacon fat until browned, then add the pesto and red pepper flakes, if using, and stir to coat. Remove the pan from the heat and cover for 5 to 10 minutes to steam the cauliflower so that it becomes tender.

2. Sprinkle with the Parmesan cheese just before serving, if desired. Store leftovers in the refrigerator for up to 3 days.

*Crazy Busy Shopping Tip:* Manufacturers like to add potato starch or canola oil to prepared pesto sauce, but not all do. Read the ingredients and look for brands that contain neither. Good ingredients include Parmesan cheese, basil, pine nuts, and olive oil. You can find prepared pesto in the refrigerated section of the grocery store or with the jarred sauces.

**Calories:** 86 | **Fat:** 6.5g | **Protein:** 3.8g | **Carbs:** 3.2g | **Fiber:** 1.3g

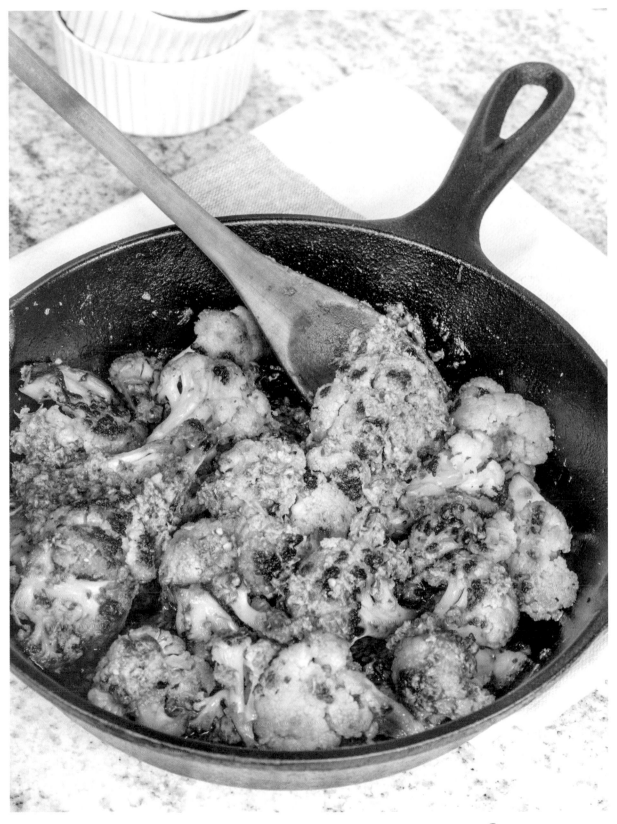

# SPEEDY CREAMED SPINACH

**MAKES** 4 servings  |  **PREP TIME:** 2 minutes  |  **COOK TIME:** 8 minutes

*You can use fresh or frozen spinach for this quick dish; both are equally fast. Arguably, fresh spinach will cook as quickly as frozen, but I used frozen spinach here because fresh spinach doesn't have a long shelf life. Frozen spinach, on the other hand, will wait for you for months to come home and cook it!*

**1 (10-ounce) package frozen spinach**

**⅓ cup heavy cream**

**2 ounces cream cheese (¼ cup)**

**2 tablespoons salted butter**

**2 tablespoons chicken broth or water (if needed)**

**1 teaspoon dried minced onion (optional)**

**¼ teaspoon garlic powder**

**¼ cup shredded Parmesan cheese**

**1.**  Cook the spinach according to the package directions. Drain and transfer to a large skillet over medium heat.

**2.**  Stir in the heavy cream, cream cheese, and butter until melted and blended. Add the broth if the mixture is too thick. Add the dried minced onion (if using) and garlic powder. Simmer over low heat for about 5 minutes, until thickened to the desired consistency.

**3.**  Remove from the heat. Sprinkle the Parmesan cheese over the spinach and serve warm. Store leftovers in the refrigerator for up to 4 days. Reheat in the microwave or on the stovetop over low heat. You may need to add an additional tablespoon of cream, broth, or water when reheating.

Calories: 174  |  Fat: 16.2g  |  Protein: 5.7g  |  Carbs: 2.2g  |  Fiber: 1.6g

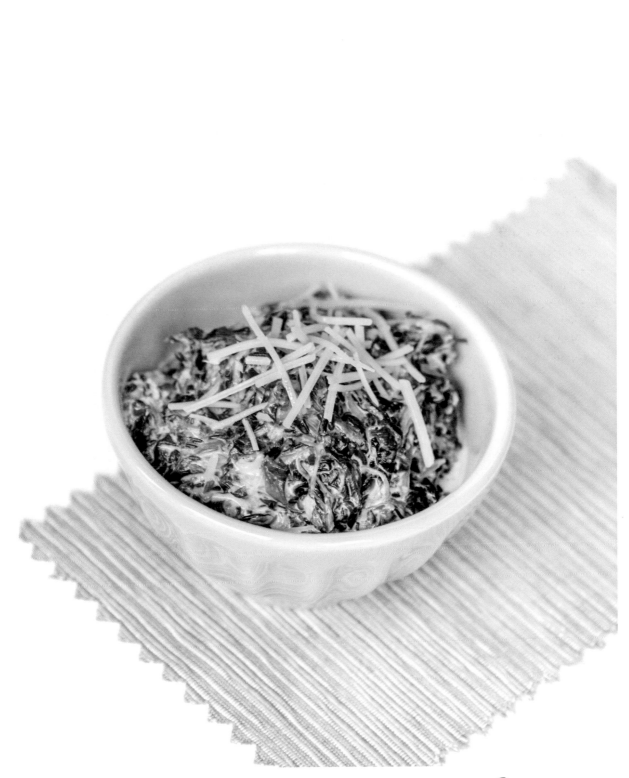

# UNSTUFFED JALAPEÑO POPPER CASSEROLE

**MAKES** 6 servings
**PREP TIME:** 6 minutes  |  **COOK TIME:** 20 minutes

*The idea for this recipe came to me one rushed weeknight when I wanted to surprise my husband with one of his favorite foods—jalapeño poppers! As I dug through the fridge, I found only a few jalapeños, some leftover mushrooms, and a bag of mini bell peppers that wouldn't last more than a few more days. I thought about stuffing them along with the jalapeños but was concerned that there wouldn't be enough time to clean and stuff each one, and then the baking times might vary. Every problem has a solution, so I decided to chop all of the veggies, mix them with the filling, and bake everything together as if it was meant to be served that way. And now it is! I serve this dish with grilled or roasted meats. It also works as a main dish that serves four since it includes protein from the sausage and cheeses.*

1 (8-ounce) package cream cheese, softened

6 ounces cheddar cheese, shredded (about 1½ cups), divided

½ teaspoon garlic powder

1 pound Italian sausage, browned and drained

4 ounces mushrooms, chopped

2 jalapeño peppers, seeded and chopped

1 cup chopped bell peppers (any color)

1 green onion, chopped, or 1 teaspoon dried chives

1. Preheat the oven to 350°F.

2. In a large bowl, mix the cream cheese, 1 cup of the cheddar cheese, and the garlic powder until well blended. Add the sausage, mushrooms, jalapeños, bell peppers, and green onion and stir to combine. The mixture will be very thick. Spoon the mixture into a 9-inch square baking dish and top with the remaining ½ cup of cheddar cheese.

3. Bake for 20 to 25 minutes, or until bubbly and lightly browned. Serve warm. Store leftovers in the refrigerator for up to 4 days. Reheat on low power in the microwave, over low heat on the stovetop, or in a low oven.

*Cook's Note:* To change things up, add cubed cooked chicken or substitute shredded cooked chicken or browned ground beef for the sausage.

Calories: 260 | Fat: 22.8g | Protein: 10.9g | Carbs: 3.9g | Fiber: 0.8g

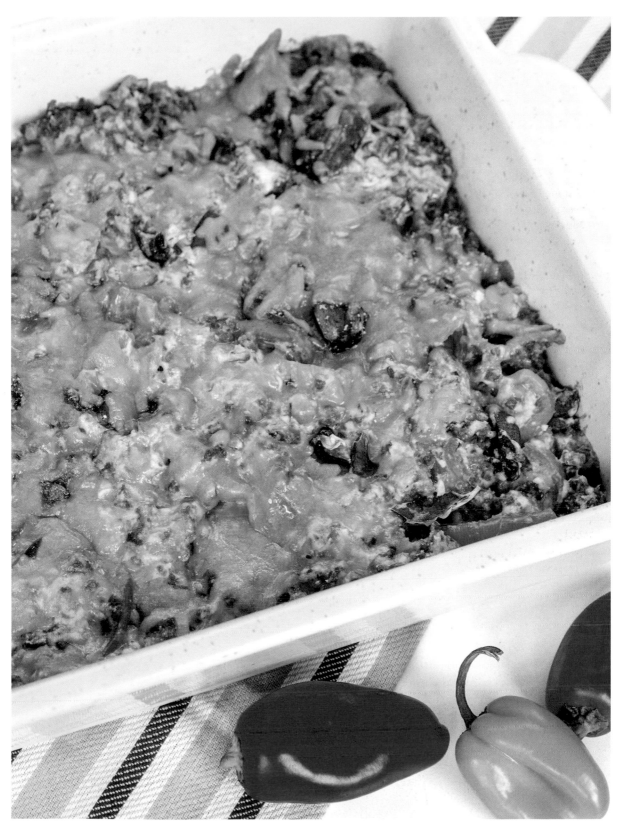

# CREAMY CUCUMBER AND RED ONION SALAD

**MAKES** 4 servings | **PREP TIME:** 4 minutes, plus 30 minutes to chill

*If every simple recipe could taste this good, life would be so much easier! We eat this salad at nearly every meal, especially in the summer. It's an easy dish to share at a potluck with minimal prep. I haven't met one person who didn't like it, and most people ask, "How do you make this?"*

½ cup sour cream

¼ cup mayonnaise

1 teaspoon white vinegar

1 teaspoon dried dill weed

¼ teaspoon salt

Dash of ground black pepper

1 large English cucumber (10 to 12 inches long), peeled and sliced

¼ cup sliced red onions

Chopped fresh dill, for garnish (optional)

1. Make the dressing: In a small bowl, stir together the sour cream, mayonnaise, vinegar, dill, salt, and pepper until combined. Set aside.

2. Use a paper towel or clean kitchen towel to pat the moisture from the cucumber slices. Place the cucumber and onion slices in a large bowl and toss to combine.

3. Pour the dressing over the cucumber and onions and toss to coat. Refrigerate for at least 30 minutes before serving. Garnish with fresh dill, if desired. Store leftovers in the refrigerator for up to 4 days.

*Cook's Note:* Don't forget to peel the cucumber; doing so reduces the carb count by about one-third!

Calories: 125 | Fat: 11g | Protein: 1.4g | Carbs: 3.9g | Fiber: 0.8g

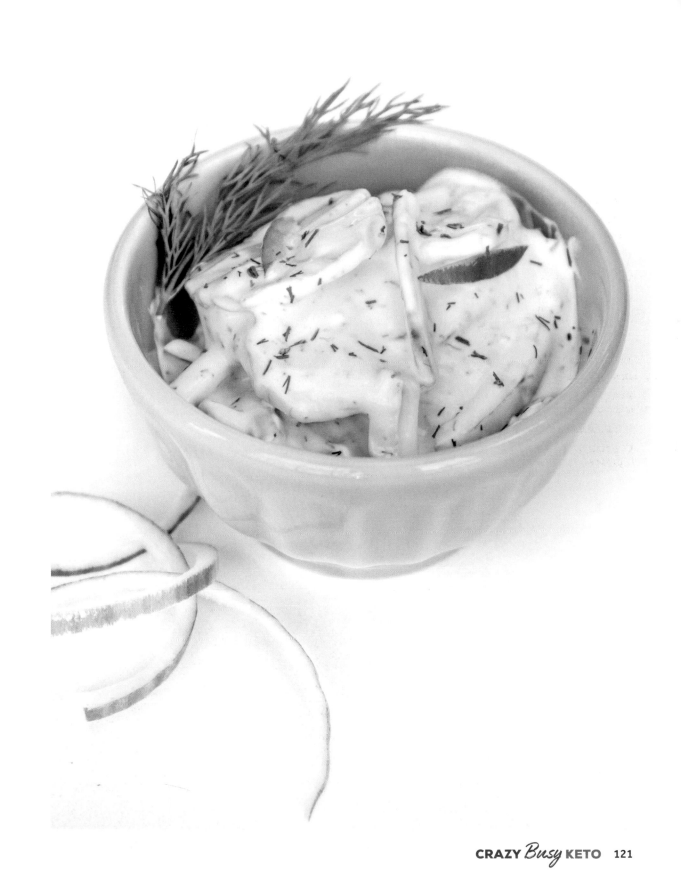

# MICROWAVED SPAGHETTI SQUASH

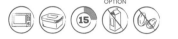

**MAKES** 8 servings (about ½ cup per serving)
**PREP TIME:** 3 minutes, plus 15 minutes to cool | **COOK TIME:** 6 minutes

*To be successful with this method of cooking spaghetti squash, you essentially stab the living daylights out of the squash, which means that you can multitask by relieving stress and fixing dinner simultaneously. Just be sure to make deep cuts in the squash so that steam can escape while it cooks. Otherwise, you will have a very stressful situation with exploded spaghetti squash coating the inside of your microwave. The squash will get very hot, so take care to use oven mitts or a towel to remove it from the microwave. Let it cool for at least 15 minutes before attempting to cut it open. This is one of those sides that I like to put in the microwave first before I begin preparing anything else so that it has time to fully cook and cool while I tend to other tasks.*

**1 medium spaghetti squash (about 3½ pounds)**

**¼ cup (½ stick) salted butter or refined coconut oil**

**1 tablespoon dried parsley (optional)**

1. Rinse and wipe dry the outside of the spaghetti squash. Use a very sharp knife to make 8 to 10 deep cuts in the squash, making sure to pierce all sides as well as the top and the bottom of the squash.

2. Microwave on full power for 6 to 8 minutes. Use an oven mitt or towel to gently squeeze the squash to check for doneness. It should yield to light pressure. Microwave for an additional minute or two if needed. Once the squash is just tender, remove it from the microwave using oven mitts or a towel and let cool for at least 15 minutes (longer is better).

3. When the squash is cool enough to handle, slice in it half lengthwise. Use a spoon to gently scrape out and discard the seeds and pulp. Scrape a fork across the flesh to loosen the spaghetti-like strands of squash. Be sure to scrape against the outer shell to release all of the flesh.

4. Toss the strands of squash with the butter and parsley, if using. Heat in the microwave or a large skillet, if needed. Serve immediately. Store leftovers in the refrigerator for up to 5 days.

> *Crazy Busy Kitchen Tip:* Microwave the squash a day ahead or in the morning on the day you want to use it. Once cool to the touch, place the whole squash in the refrigerator. When you're ready to use it, complete Steps 3 and 4.

**Calories:** 51 | **Fat:** 5.8g | **Protein:** 0.1g | **Carbs:** 2g | **Fiber:** 0.2g

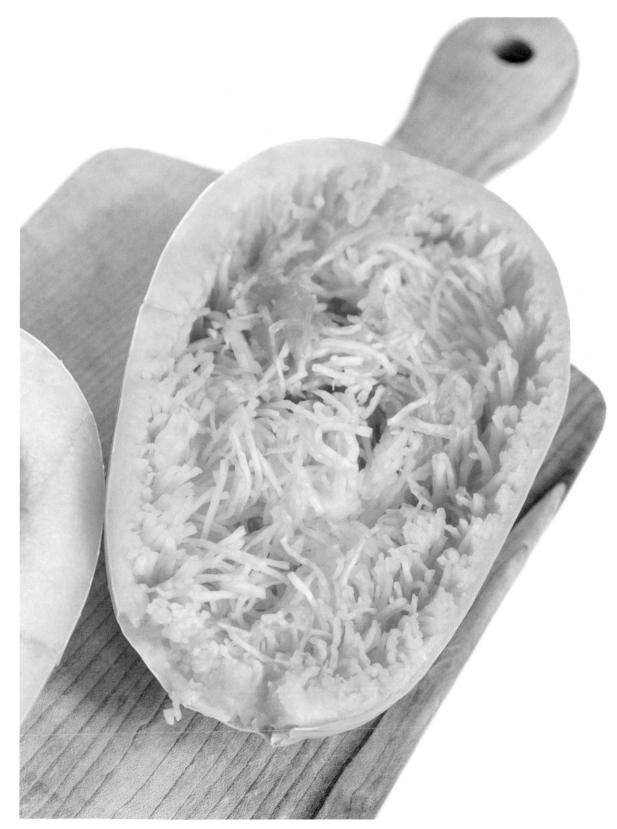

# MEXICAN FIESTA CAULI RICE

OPTION

(15)

**MAKES** 6 servings (about ⅓ cup per serving)
**PREP TIME:** 5 minutes | **COOK TIME:** 8 minutes

*The colors of this dish make it look festive, tempting the eyes and hinting at the burst of flavor in every bite! This is no ordinary cauli rice. This dish dresses up plain frozen riced cauliflower so that you can take it anywhere. Enjoy it as a side dish paired with seasoned ground beef or shredded cooked chicken, or scoop a smaller portion into Nachos Two Ways (page 60). Because this recipe uses small amounts of a variety of veggies, it's a great example of a meal you can make from the grocery salad bar (see page 8), saving you time and money. If you don't have time to seed and dice a fresh jalapeño, you can use 1 tablespoon of diced jarred jalapeño instead.*

1 tablespoon bacon fat

½ cup diced bell peppers (any color)

⅓ cup chopped red onions

1 jalapeño pepper, seeded and diced

6 grape tomatoes, chopped

2 tablespoons salted butter or refined coconut oil

¼ teaspoon dried cilantro (aka coriander leaf)

⅛ teaspoon garlic powder

⅛ teaspoon ground cumin

1 (10-ounce) package frozen riced cauliflower

Grated zest of 1 lime (optional)

Juice of 1 lime (about 2 tablespoons)

¼ teaspoon salt

Fresh cilantro leaves, for garnish (optional)

1. Heat the bacon fat in a large skillet over medium-high heat. Add the peppers, onions, and jalapeño and sauté in the bacon fat for 4 to 6 minutes, or until crisp-tender.

2. Reduce the heat to medium-low and stir in the tomatoes, butter, dried cilantro, garlic powder, and cumin. Add the cauliflower and allow to thaw in the skillet with the pepper mixture.

3. When the cauliflower is thawed, stir in the lime zest (if using), lime juice, and salt. Serve immediately, garnished with fresh cilantro leaves, if desired. Store leftovers in the refrigerator for up to 3 days and enjoy cold or warmed in the microwave.

Calories: 89 | Fat: 6.5g | Protein: 1.7g | Carbs: 5.4g | Fiber: 2.2g

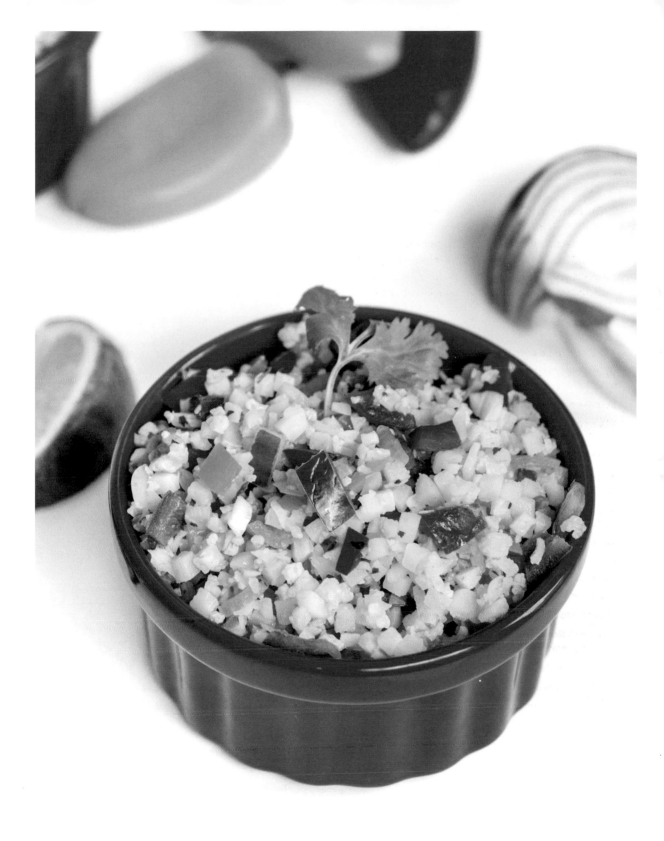

# LOADED BAKED YELLOW SQUASH

**MAKES** 2 servings | **PREP TIME:** 3 minutes, plus 5 minutes to cool (not including time to cook bacon if not purchased precooked) | **COOK TIME:** 3 minutes

*Remember how you used to microwave a "baked" potato? This recipe follows the same principle, except you're using a yellow squash instead! Even better, yellow squash is truly low-carb. Most small summer squash weigh less than a pound and cook quickly, which makes this a super simple and inexpensive side dish with minimal cleanup. Adding butter, bacon, sour cream, and cheese makes it an easy staple that you can also enjoy while traveling. A smaller squash works best because it will have smaller seeds and more edible flesh.*

1 small yellow summer squash
(about 12 ounces)

2 tablespoons unsalted butter

1⅓ ounces cheddar cheese,
shredded (about ⅓ cup)

¼ cup crumbled cooked bacon

2 tablespoons sour cream

1 tablespoon sliced green onions,
for garnish (optional)

1. Wash the squash and wipe it dry. Use a sharp knife to piece the flesh of the squash at least six times, making random cuts on all sides.

2. Wrap the squash in a damp paper towel. Microwave on full power for 3 to 4 minutes. The squash is done when it yields to slight pressure.

3. Use a towel or oven mitt to remove the squash from the microwave. Let cool for 5 to 10 minutes, then slice it open lengthwise. Fill the halves with equal amounts of the butter, cheese, and bacon. Top with the sour cream just before serving. Garnish with sliced green onions, if desired.

*Cook's Note:* If you won't be consuming both servings of the loaded squash right away, reserve half of the sour cream and onions to place on the leftover portion after reheating.

Calories: 216 | Fat: 20.6g | Protein: 6.1g | Carbs: 2.8g | Fiber: 0.7g

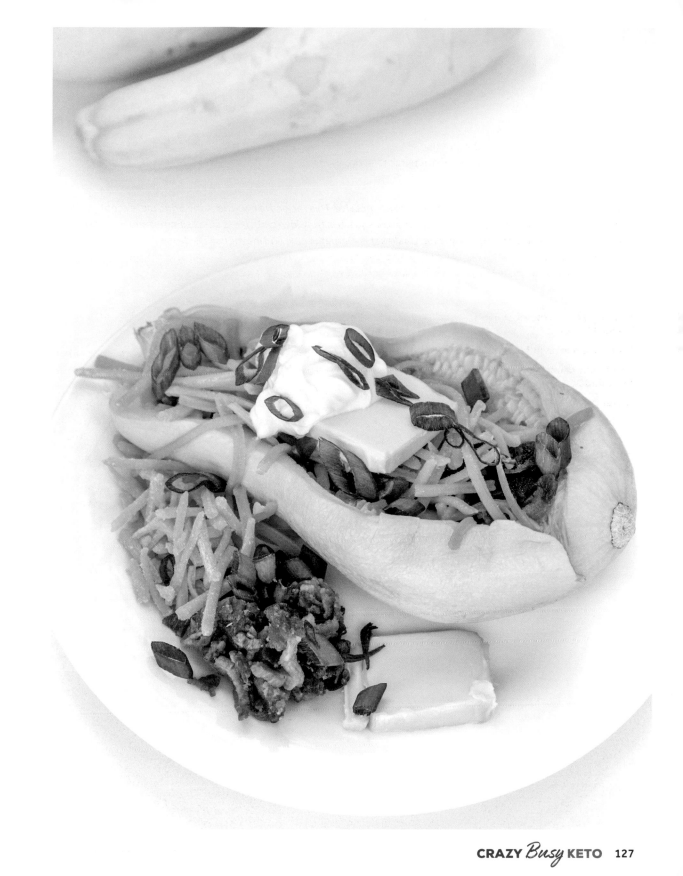

# CREAMY AVOCADO SALSA

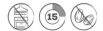

**MAKES** 1¼ cups (about ¼ cup per serving)
**PREP TIME:** 3 minutes

*Avocados won't wait for you to go to the store and buy fresh cilantro and tomatoes. This quick recipe is the solution: it uses prepared salsa and dried cilantro (aka coriander leaf). Dried cilantro doesn't wilt! That said, you can use 2 tablespoons of chopped fresh cilantro in its place if you have it. We enjoy this salsa as a quick side with any Southwestern-style main dish that includes seasoned taco meat, such as chicken or ground beef, or even cooked Mexican-style (fresh) chorizo.*

**1 ripe avocado, chopped**

**½ cup sour cream**

**⅓ cup prepared salsa**

**1 teaspoon dried cilantro (aka coriander leaf)**

**1 teaspoon lime juice (optional)**

Mix all the ingredients together in a small bowl. Store leftover salsa in the refrigerator for up to 3 days.

*Crazy Busy Shopping Tips:* When buying prepared salsa, look for brands without added sugars or food starches such as dextrose or maltodextrin, and avoid those products that contain canola or soybean oil.

*Also, store-brand sour cream often has more fat and less carbs than popular brands.*

Calories: 113 | Fat: 10.6g | Protein: 1.5g | Carbs: 2.4g | Fiber: 1.7g

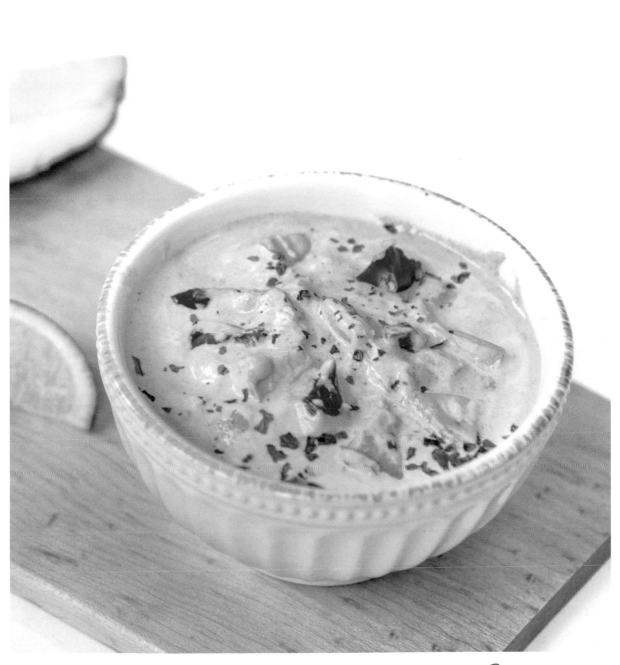

# FETA CREAM SAUCE

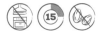

**MAKES** 2 servings (about ⅓ cup per serving)
**PREP TIME:** 3 minutes

*This quick sauce is great with grilled meats and can be used to liven up canned tuna, shrimp, or chicken. While it's best if chilled for at least 30 minutes before eating, it can be made and served immediately. It makes an excellent dip for the Greek Wings on page 72.*

½ cup sour cream

2 ounces feta cheese, crumbled (about ½ cup)

1 tablespoon lemon juice

1 teaspoon dried minced onion

½ teaspoon dried oregano leaves

4 Kalamata olives, pitted and chopped (optional)

Grated lemon zest, for garnish (optional)

Mix all the ingredients together in a small bowl. If time allows, refrigerate the sauce for at least 30 minutes before serving. Garnish with grated lemon zest, if desired. Store leftover sauce in the refrigerator for up to 4 days.

*Cook's Notes:* You can use a feta cheese flavored with basil or sun-dried tomatoes if you like. Also, if you don't care for the strong taste of feta, you can substitute fresh goat cheese, which is generally much milder but has a similar texture.

**Calories:** 202 | **Fat:** 18.2g | **Protein:** 6g | **Carbs:** 3.4g | **Fiber:** 0.6g

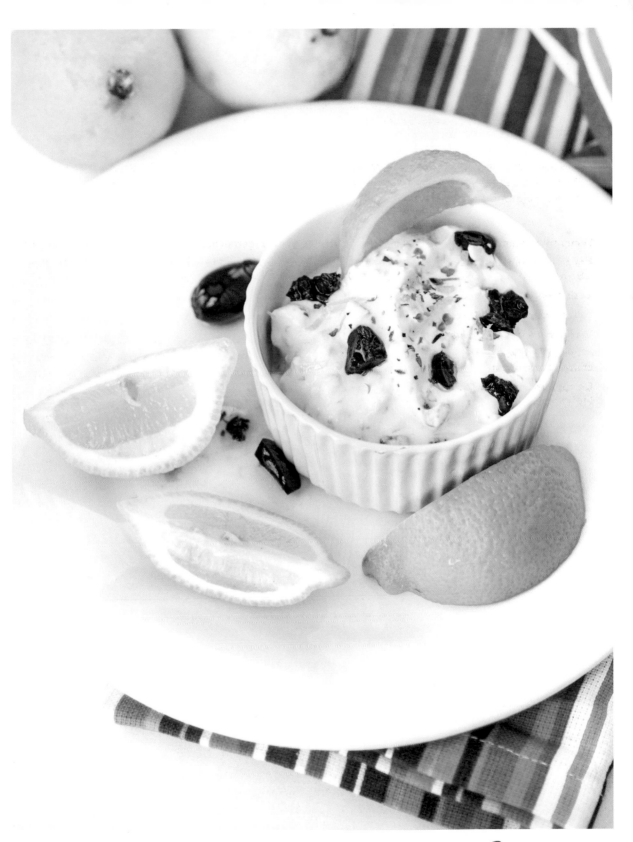

# TZATZIKI SAUCE

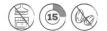

**MAKES** 6 servings (about ¼ cup per serving)
**PREP TIME:** 8 minutes, plus 30 minutes to chill

*Zat-zee-key—it's fun to say and even more fun to eat! Whether you're enjoying it with Greek Wings (page 72), Greek Meatballs (page 88), or peeled and sliced cucumbers, it's as refreshing and light as the sunshine on a Greek island. This is one of my favorite sauces to pair with any grilled meat, especially lamb or chicken.*

1¼ cups sour cream

½ cup peeled, seeded, and finely chopped cucumber, drained

1 tablespoon lemon juice

1 teaspoon minced garlic

1 teaspoon dried minced onion, or 2 teaspoons finely chopped red onions

1 teaspoon ground cumin

1 teaspoon dried dill weed

½ teaspoon salt

Chopped fresh dill or parsley, for garnish

Mix all the ingredients together in a small bowl. Refrigerate for at least 30 minutes before serving. Garnish with fresh dill. Store leftover sauce in the refrigerator for up to 5 days.

Calories: 133 | Fat: 16g | Protein: 3.5g | Carbs: 3.2g | Fiber: 0.6g

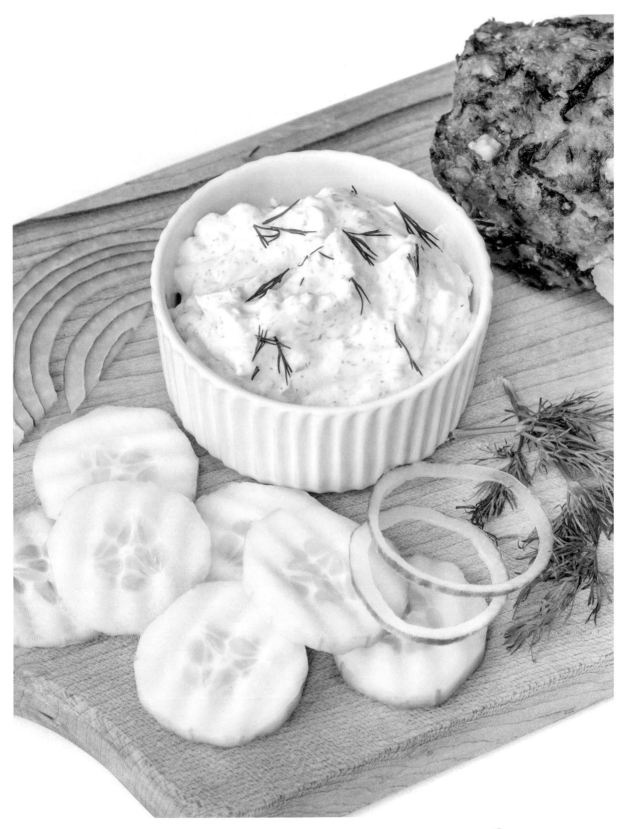

# THAI PEANUT SAUCE

**MAKES** about 2½ cups (⅓ cup per serving)
**PREP TIME:** 3 minutes | **COOK TIME:** 4 minutes

*This is one of those sauces that can make shoe leather taste good! My favorite use for it is the Thai Chicken Slaw recipe on page 84, but it's great with any grilled meat, veggie "noodles," or a simple salad. You can thin the sauce with a little more coconut milk or even chicken broth if you find it too thick. The sauce does thin when heated.*

1 (13½-ounce) can full-fat coconut milk

⅓ cup creamy peanut butter (salted, unsweetened)

¼ cup coconut aminos or tamari

2 tablespoons fish sauce (omit if using tamari)

2 tablespoons unseasoned rice wine vinegar

2 tablespoons toasted sesame oil

1 tablespoon minced fresh ginger

1 tablespoon minced garlic

¼ teaspoon cayenne pepper (optional)

4 drops liquid sweetener (optional)

Place the coconut milk and peanut butter in a medium-sized heavy saucepan over low heat and stir until the peanut butter is melted and the ingredients are well blended. Stir in the remaining ingredients and continue stirring until the sauce comes to a low simmer, then remove from the heat. Use warm or cold as a sauce or salad dressing. Store leftover sauce in the refrigerator for up to 1 week.

Calories: 253 | Fat: 23.2g | Protein: 6.3g | Carbs: 4.9g | Fiber: 1.8g

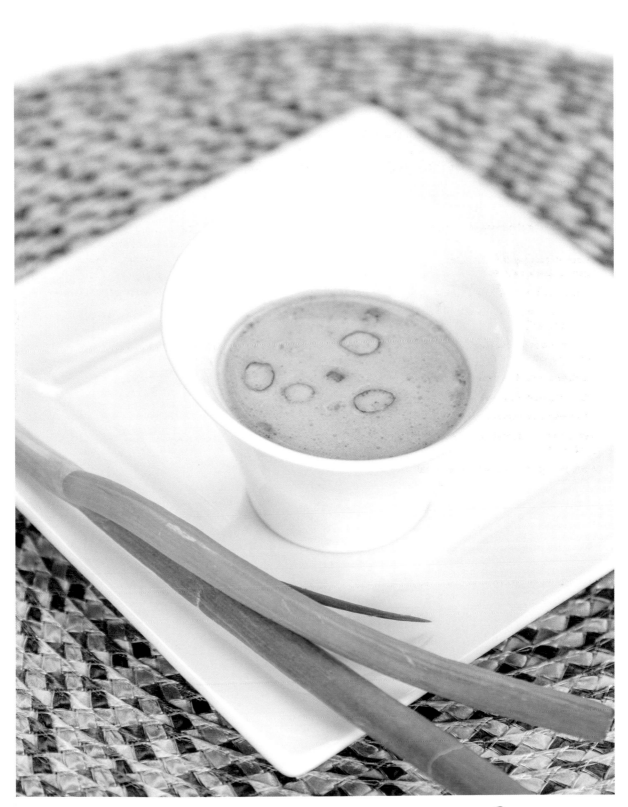

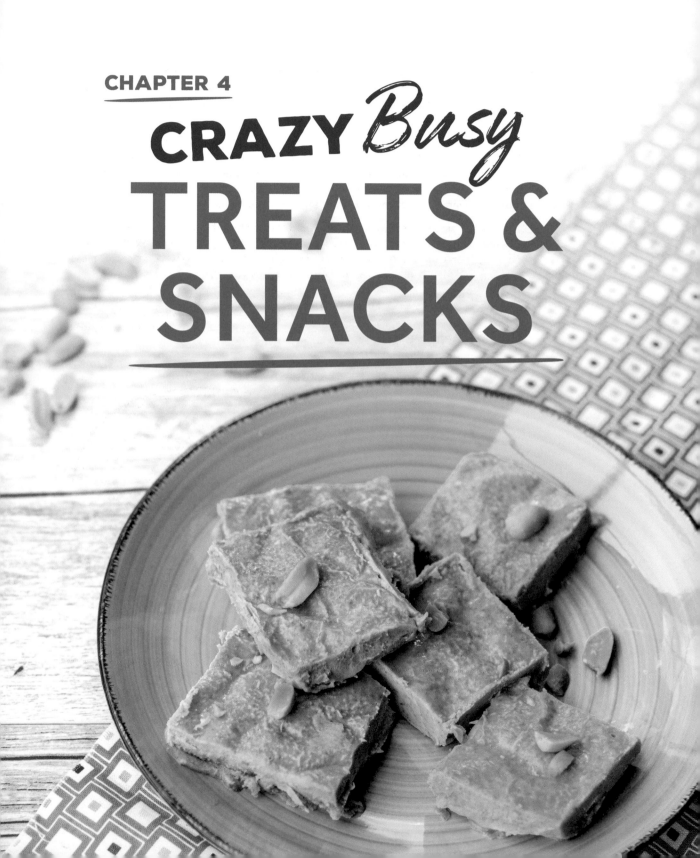

# CHAPTER 4

# CRAZY *Busy*
# TREATS & SNACKS

Even though most of us don't snack on keto because we aren't hungry between meals, it's nice to have options when you need them. The ideas and recipes included in this chapter were designed to be made quickly and travel well. Some of them will satisfy your sweet tooth if it gets loud.

Without a doubt, two of my favorite recipes in this chapter are the Cheesecake in Minutes and the Chili-Lime Trail Mix. First, I really like that the cheesecake recipe makes two portions, doesn't require an oven, and can be made anywhere you have access to a microwave. Even though this cheesecake has to be refrigerated for several hours before serving, the texture rivals a traditional oven-baked cheesecake that's much fussier to make.

The trail mix is a favorite because it's portable, resembles a high-carb snack, and has an amazing flavor. It's an exception to the other quick recipes in this chapter because it takes a while to bake, but you can busy yourself with other tasks while the oven does most of the work. After the mix is done, you simply bag it up, and there's nothing more to do than enjoy it.

I've noted which of these treats can be frozen and which travel well, but I haven't noted which ones you might want to share, because that's entirely up to you. Still, I can assure you that my friends and family have taste-tested all of these recipes, and I wouldn't hesitate to share any of them with others, whether they follow keto or not.

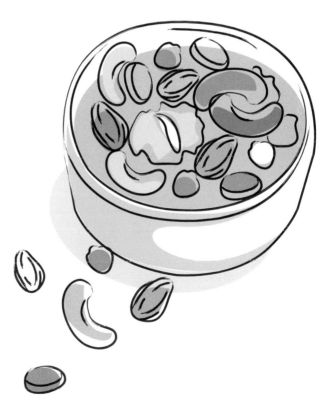

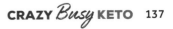

# -SNACK *Ideas*-

## CHEESE CRACKER SNACKS

To make these little cracker snacks super simple, I buy premade Parmesan chips, aka "cheese crisps," that are easily found in grocery stores and warehouse stores. In particular, I like the small round Parmesan crisps (for suggested brands, see page 160). Parmesan cheese crisps are a standout as fantastic little snack treats, especially when spread with keto BFFs like butter, cream cheese, almond butter, or peanut butter.

*Cook's Note:* While you can make these cheese cracker snacks ahead of time, they are best consumed within 4 to 5 hours of making if you want them to stay crisp. After several hours, the crisps will absorb the moisture from the filling and may become a bit soft.

## PEANUT BUTTER (OR ALMOND BUTTER) SANDWICH CRACKERS

Before keto, I used to eat peanut butter cheese crackers at least once per day. Truthfully, more often than that. Those six-packs of crackers were a single-serving snack to me. I hadn't missed them very much after starting keto until a friend gave me the idea to put a smear of peanut butter on a Parmesan cheese crisp. One bite took me right back to those high-carb favorites! You can also use almond butter if you avoid legumes. To make, have on hand 24 small Parmesan cheese crisps (about the size of a quarter) and about 1 tablespoon of unsweetened peanut butter or almond butter. Smear a dollop of peanut butter about the size of a pea on one of the cheese crisps. Top with a second cheese crisp. Repeat until 12 sandwiches are made.

## BUTTER SANDWICH CRACKERS

Have on hand 24 small Parmesan cheese crisps (about the size of a quarter) and about 1½ tablespoons of unsalted butter at room temperature. Coat one side of a cracker with a thick layer of butter. Top with a second cheese crisp. Repeat until 12 sandwiches are made.

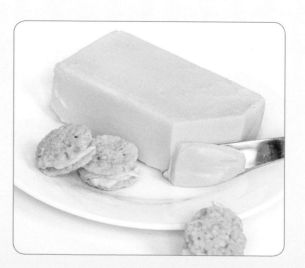

## CREAM CHEESE SANDWICH CRACKERS

Have on hand 24 small Parmesan cheese crisps (about the size of a quarter) and 1 ounce of cream cheese, softened. Smear a thick layer of cream cheese on one side of a Parmesan cheese crisp, about ¼ inch thick. Top with a second cheese crisp. Repeat until 12 sandwiches are made.

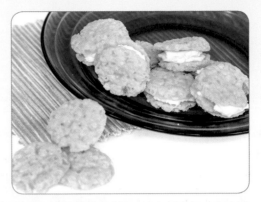

## ALMOND BUTTER BOOST

Although there are a few good commercial nut butter options, it's worth making this treat. It's super simple, inexpensive, and easy to eat on the road. All you need is a spoon and a small cup or bowl. You can also mix the ingredients ahead of time in small condiment cups and have them ready to drop into a bag, purse, or lunch box. They make a quick snack or supplement to a meal that needs more fat. They also provide a way to enjoy nut butter in moderation while adding fat and reducing the overall carb count by stretching the flavor. Peanut butter or any other nut butter can be used instead of the almond butter.

**1 tablespoon almond butter (unsweetened)**

**1 tablespoon salted butter or refined coconut oil, softened**

**Dash of ground cinnamon**

**Dash of salt**

**Drop of liquid sweetener (optional)**

Mix all the ingredients in a small bowl until well blended. Store at room temperature for up to 5 days.

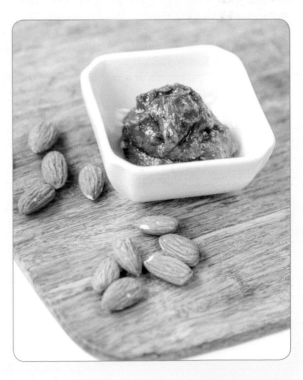

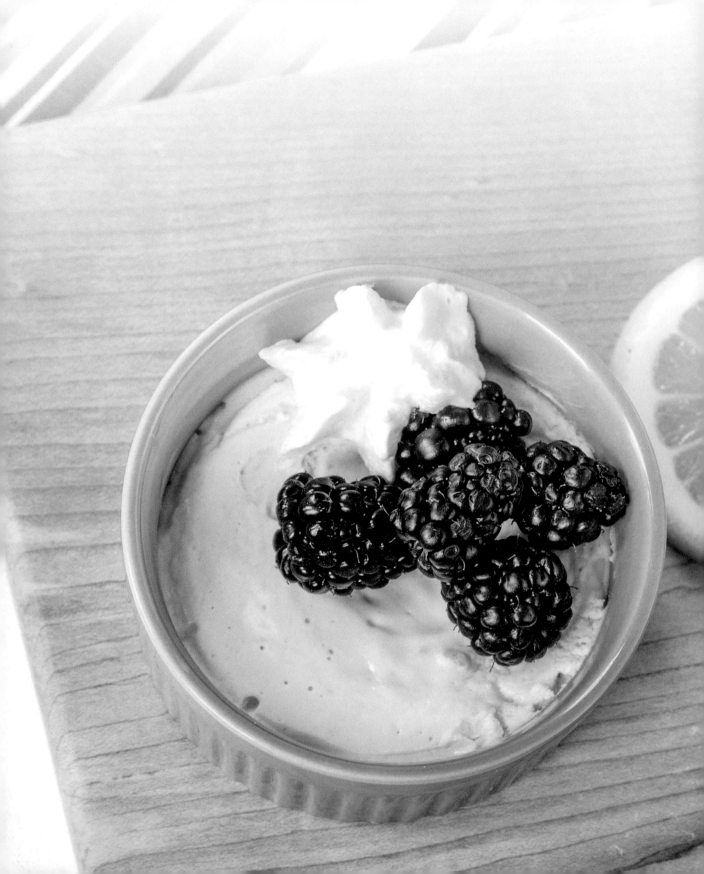

# Recipes

# STRAWBERRY CREAM PIE

**MAKES** 8 servings | **PREP TIME:** 14 minutes, plus 4 hours to chill

*Before going low-carb, I made this pie with a store-bought graham cracker crust and real sugar. It was easy to create a low-carb version, and I love that I can have it chilling in the fridge in less than 15 minutes. The difficult part is waiting for it to set up. My husband prefers the filling served without the crust in a small parfait glass or dessert dish.*

**FILLING:**

**1 (8-ounce) package cream cheese, slightly softened**

**½ cup powdered sweetener**

**1 tablespoon lemon juice**

**2 teaspoons vanilla extract**

**1 teaspoon strawberry extract (optional)**

**1¼ cups heavy cream**

**1 cup thinly sliced strawberries, plus 4 extra strawberries for garnish if desired**

**CRUST:**

**¾ cup blanched almond flour**

**3 tablespoons granulated sweetener**

**1 tablespoon unsalted butter, melted**

**¼ teaspoon salt**

1.  Take the cream cheese for the filling out of the fridge about 20 minutes before making the recipe; it needs to have the chill taken off it but does not need to be fully softened.

2.  Make the crust: Place all the ingredients for the crust in a small bowl or a food processor and mix with a spatula or the food processor until they resemble coarse crumbs. Press the mixture across the bottom and up the sides of a 9-inch pie pan to form a crust. Set aside.

3.  Make the filling: In a large bowl, whip the cream cheese with a hand mixer until creamy. Add the powdered sweetener, lemon juice, and extracts and continue to whip until smooth. Pour in the heavy cream in three parts, blending well after each addition. When the mixture is whipped and fluffy, stir in the sliced berries by hand.

4.  Smooth the filling into the prepared crust. If using extra strawberries for garnish, slice them and arrange them on top of the pie as you like. Refrigerate the pie for at least 4 hours or overnight before serving. Store leftovers in the refrigerator for up to 4 days.

**Calories:** 320 | **Fat:** 31.9g | **Protein:** 3.9g | **Carbs:** 4.8g | **Fiber:** 1.9g | **Erythritol:** 18g

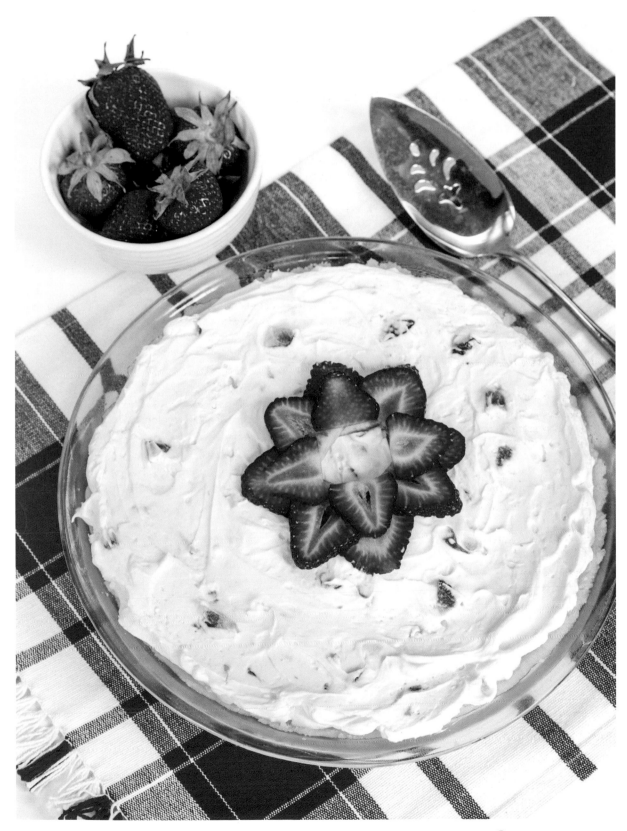

# CHEESECAKE IN MINUTES

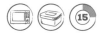

**MAKES** 2 servings
**PREP TIME:** 2 minutes, plus 8½ hours to cool and chill  |  **COOK TIME:** 3½ minutes

*The good news is that this recipe takes only minutes to put together and "bake" in the microwave. The bad news is that, like any cheesecake, it needs to chill and "cure" for at least eight hours, which is God's way of telling us that cheesecake for breakfast is perfectly acceptable. The better news is that it's nicely low in carbs and perfectly legal on your keto diet!*

*Be sure to microwave the cheesecakes on reduced power so that they don't overcook and the texture remains similar to baked cheesecake. If you prefer, you can bake them in a regular oven at 325°F for 18 to 22 minutes, or until just set in the center. Using two egg yolks gives the cheesecakes a creamier texture, but you can use one whole egg if you prefer.*

**¼ cup blanched almond flour**

**½ tablespoon unsalted butter, melted**

**4 ounces cream cheese (½ cup), softened**

**3 tablespoons granulated sweetener**

**¼ cup sour cream**

**1 teaspoon vanilla extract**

**1 teaspoon lemon juice**

**2 large egg yolks, or 1 whole large egg**

### TOPPINGS (OPTIONAL):

**Whipped cream**

**Fresh berries of choice**

1.  Grease two microwave-safe 8-ounce ramekins or coffee mugs. In a small bowl, combine the almond flour and melted butter to make a crust. The mixture will be coarse. Divide the crust mixture evenly between the ramekins and press firmly into the bottom.

2.  In another bowl, use a hand mixer to whip the cream cheese and sweetener until smooth and creamy. Add the sour cream, vanilla extract, and lemon juice and mix until blended and creamy. Use a rubber spatula to mix in the egg yolks. Divide the batter evenly between the ramekins, pouring it over the crusts.

3.  Microwave both ramekins together at 50% power for 1 minute. Continue to microwave at 50% power in 20- to 30-second increments until the cheesecakes begin to set. It may take an additional 2½ to 3½ minutes of incremental heating. Remove from the microwave when the centers are still a bit wet or shiny. Do not overcook; the cheesecakes will continue to firm up as they cool.

4.  Let cool at room temperature for about 30 minutes before covering and refrigerating for at least 8 hours; the cheesecakes will have the best consistency if left to chill overnight. If desired, top with whipped cream and/or berries before serving. Store leftovers in the fridge for up to 1 week. Individual cheesecakes also freeze well.

> *Cook's Notes: While in the microwave, the tops of the cheesecakes should stay smooth. If the tops or sides begin to bubble, cook for no longer than 20 seconds per burst of heat rather than 30 seconds.*
>
> *My microwave has 1250 watts. If yours has a lower wattage, you may need to increase the cooking time a bit.*

Calories: 425 | Fat: 40.2g | Protein: 8.9g | Carbs: 3.1g | Fiber: 1.5g | Erythritol: 12g

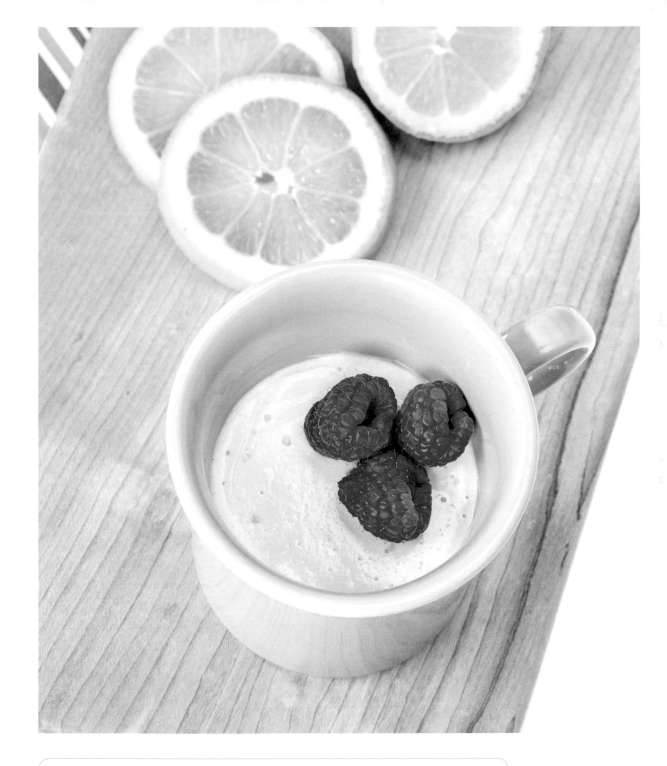

*Crazy Busy Travel Tip:* If you only have access to a microwave and a fridge, you can still make this dessert! You will need to find microwave-safe coffee cups, something to use as a mixing bowl, and a sturdy fork to make the cheesecake filling.

# CHILI-LIME TRAIL MIX

**MAKES** 8 cups (⅔ cup per serving)
**PREP TIME:** 8 minutes, plus 1½ hours to cool | **COOK TIME:** 1½ hours

*While I never share a recipe I don't like, this recipe is one of my absolute favorites. I'm proud of the way the flavors came together, and I'm proud of the combination of ingredients that makes it low enough in carbs that you can have a good-sized portion. This could easily be a meal on the road, tucked into lunches, or sneaked into a movie theater.*

**3 tablespoons chili powder**

**2 teaspoons salt**

**½ teaspoon cayenne pepper**

**½ teaspoon garlic powder**

**½ teaspoon onion powder**

**3 cups Parmesan cheese crisps, broken into bite-sized pieces**

**3 cups broken pork rind pieces (about 1½ ounces)**

**1 cup raw peanuts**

**½ cup raw almonds, chopped**

**½ cup raw cashew pieces**

**½ cup raw pecan pieces**

**¼ cup raw pumpkin seeds**

**1 large egg white**

**3½ tablespoons lime juice**

1. Preheat the oven to 200°F. Line a rimmed baking sheet with parchment paper or aluminum foil, then lightly grease the paper or foil and set aside.

2. In a small bowl or cup, mix together the chili powder, salt, cayenne pepper, garlic powder, and onion powder. In a large bowl, combine the cheese crisps, pork rind pieces, peanuts, almonds, cashews, pecans, and pumpkin seeds.

3. In a separate small bowl, whisk the egg white until frothy. Add the lime juice and continue whisking until blended and frothy.

4. Pour the egg white mixture over the nut mixture and toss to thoroughly coat each piece. Sprinkle the seasoning mixture over the trail mix, stirring so that each piece is seasoned.

5. Spread the trail mix in a single layer on the prepared baking sheet. Bake for 25 minutes, then use a spatula to stir. Continue baking, giving the trail mix a gentle stir every 15 to 20 minutes, until it is lightly browned and crisp; the total cooking time will be about 1½ hours. When the trail mix is crisp, turn the oven off, open the oven door slightly, turn on the oven light, and leave it to cool for at least 1½ hours or overnight. The trail mix will become crisper as it sits in the oven with the light on.

6. Remove from the oven and let cool to room temperature. Store in an airtight container in the refrigerator for up to 2 weeks.

Calories: 298 | Fat: 28.2g | Protein: 26g | Carbs: 6.4g | Fiber: 3.1g

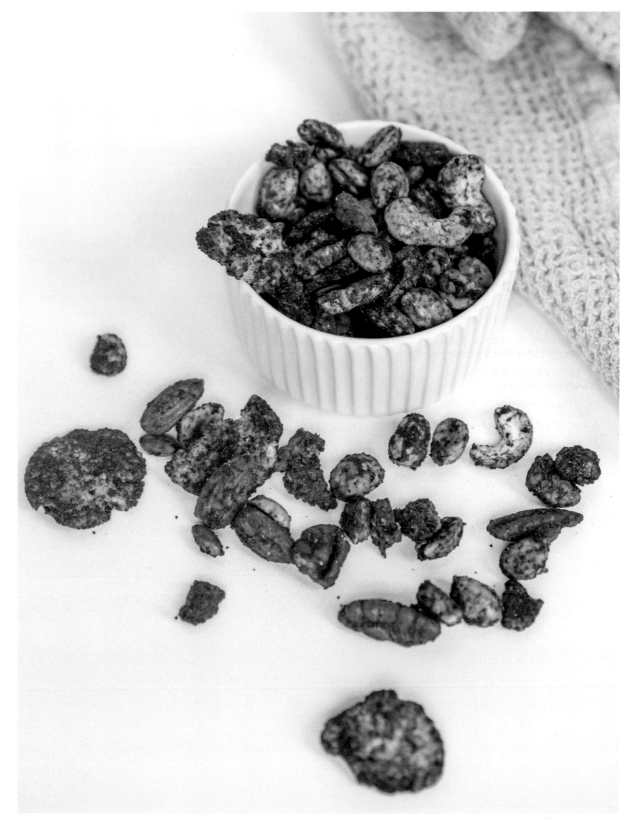

# FORGOTTEN COOKIES

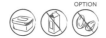

**MAKES** 18 cookies (3 per serving)
**PREP TIME:** 6 minutes, plus overnight to cool | **COOK TIME:** 1 hour

*I've always avoided making cookies because preparing and portioning the dough and then baking it can be pretty time-consuming. Even while baking, the cookies need to be watched carefully. These cookies are different—they thrive on being "forgotten"! You mix them, drop them, put them in the oven, turn off the oven, and forget them overnight. When you come back to them, they will be unforgettable!*

2 large egg whites, room temperature

⅛ teaspoon cream of tartar

⅛ teaspoon salt

2 tablespoons powdered sweetener

1 teaspoon vanilla extract

2 tablespoons chopped raw pecans (optional)

1 tablespoon low-carb chocolate chips or chopped dark chocolate (90% cacao)

1. Preheat the oven to 225°F. Line a rimmed baking sheet with parchment paper or a silicone baking mat. Generously grease the paper or mat.

2. In a clean metal or glass bowl, use a hand mixer to whip the egg whites, cream of tartar, and salt until foamy. Add the sweetener gradually while continuing to whip. Pour in the vanilla extract and keep whipping until stiff peaks form. Use a rubber spatula to fold in the nuts, if using, and the chocolate.

3. Using a small cookie scoop or a large spoon, drop the mixture onto the prepared baking sheet, spacing the cookies at least ½ inch apart. Bake for 1 hour. After an hour, turn off the oven but do not open the oven door. Let the cookies sit in the oven with the door closed overnight before serving. Store leftovers in an airtight container at room temperature for up to 5 days.

> *Cook's Note:* If you omit both the nuts and the chocolate, you can pipe the dough onto the baking sheet to make meringue cookies, but who has time for that?

Calories: 8 | Fat: 0g | Protein: 1.2g | Carbs: 0.2g | Fiber: 0g | Erythritol: 8g

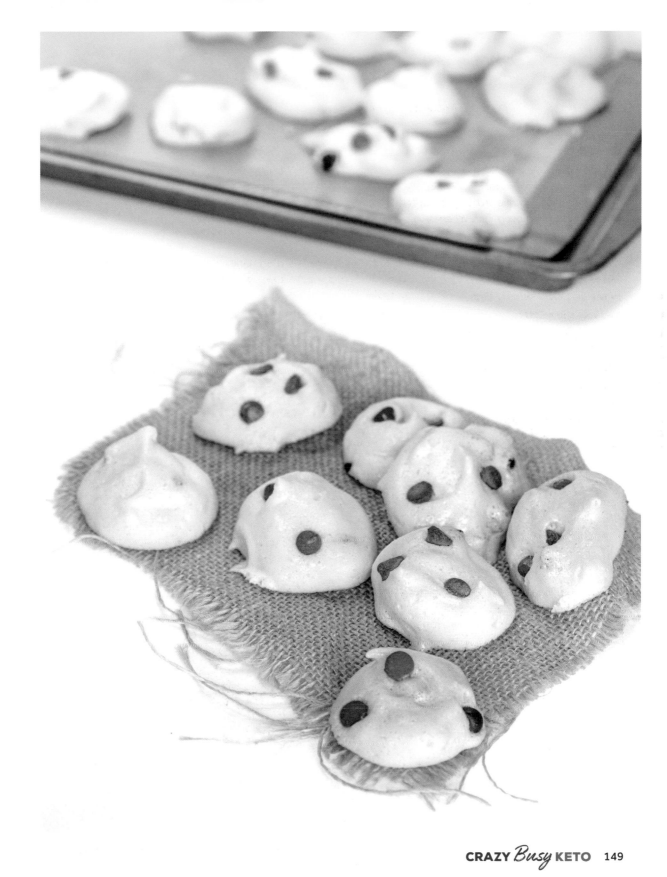

# WHIPPED CHEESECAKE DREAM

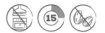

**MAKES** 4 servings  |  **PREP TIME:** 6 minutes, plus 1 hour to chill

*My daughter and husband sometimes make this treat when I'm away or just too busy. They tend to get heavy-handed with the lemon juice, as they like it super lemony. I prefer less lemon so that it tastes a little more like cheesecake. You can also add low-carb chocolate chips or omit the lemon juice and add ¼ cup of peanut butter and a dash or two of salt.*

**1 (8-ounce) package cream cheese, softened**

**⅓ cup powdered sweetener**

**½ cup sour cream**

**¼ cup heavy cream**

**1 tablespoon vanilla extract**

**1 tablespoon lemon juice**

**¼ teaspoon salt**

**Grated lemon zest, for garnish (optional)**

1.  Place the cream cheese and sweetener in a medium bowl and use a hand mixer to blend until the sweetener is dissolved. Whip in the sour cream and heavy cream. Add the vanilla extract, lemon juice, and salt and stir by hand to combine.

2.  Divide the cheesecake among four 4-ounce serving dishes. Refrigerate for at least 1 hour before serving. Garnish with grated lemon zest, if desired. Store leftovers in the refrigerator for up to 4 days.

**Calories:** 296 | **Fat:** 28.6g | **Protein:** 5.4g | **Carbs:** 3.4g | **Fiber:** 0g | **Erythritol:** 24g

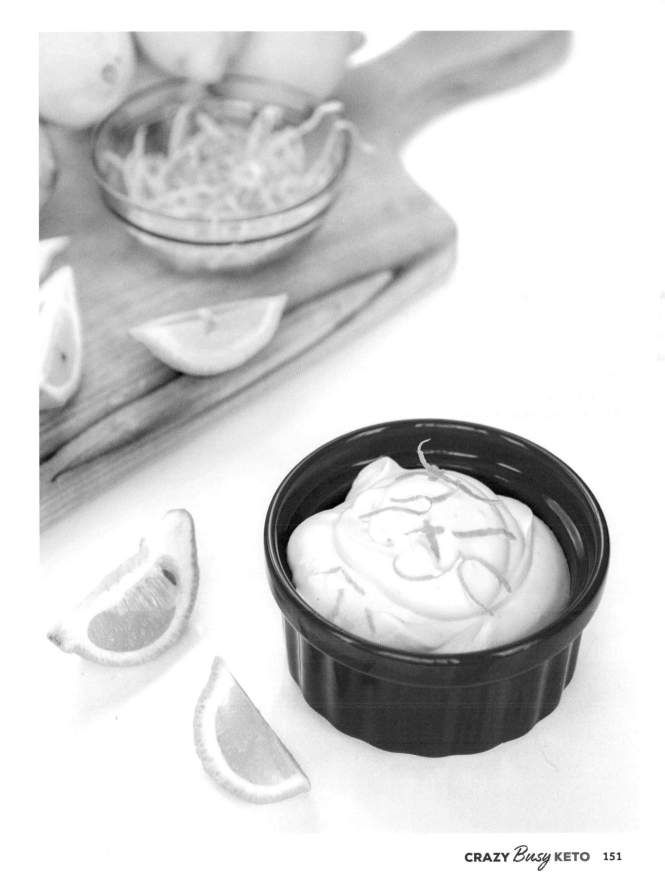

# PEANUT BUTTER FUDGE

**MAKES** 9 servings
**PREP TIME:** 3 minutes, plus 4 hours to chill | **COOK TIME:** 7 minutes

*This fudge has gotten me through many days when I didn't have time to stop for lunch. Although it doesn't have enough protein to be considered a good lunch option, it is an option. However, the fudge really does need to be refrigerated, as it becomes very soft even at room temperature. I prefer to store it in the freezer, which helps with portion control. Plus, when you take a small bite from a frozen piece of fudge, it tends to melt more slowly in your mouth. Be patient when simmering the heavy cream and powdered sweetener. It takes time to thicken to the right consistency, which should be similar to that of sweetened condensed milk. Also, be sure to take the pan off the heat before adding the butter and coconut oil. The butter and coconut oil need just enough heat to melt them; if the mixture is too warm, it will separate.*

1¼ cups heavy cream

½ cup powdered sweetener

1 cup creamy peanut butter (salted, unsweetened)

½ cup (1 stick) salted butter

⅓ cup refined coconut oil

2 teaspoons vanilla extract

½ teaspoon ground cinnamon (optional)

¼ teaspoon salt

2 tablespoons roughly chopped roasted and salted peanuts, for garnish (optional)

1. Bring the heavy cream to a low simmer in a medium-sized heavy saucepan over low heat. Whisk in the sweetener until dissolved. Simmer for 10 to 12 minutes, or until reduced and thickened to the consistency of sweetened condensed milk.

2. Remove the pan from the heat, then stir in the peanut butter, butter, and coconut oil until melted and creamy. Add the remaining ingredients and stir well. Let cool for 10 to 15 minutes, then pour the mixture into an 8-inch square baking dish and refrigerate for at least 4 hours.

3. Cut into squares and serve. Garnish with the chopped peanuts just before serving, if desired. The fudge becomes very soft at room temperature, so it is best kept chilled. Store leftovers in the refrigerator for up to 1 week or in the freezer for up to 2 months.

*Cook's Note:* If you don't care for the flavor of coconut oil, use an extra ⅓ cup of salted butter instead. You may not need to add the ¼ teaspoon of salt.

**Calories:** 205 | **Fat:** 20.9g | **Protein:** 3.8g | **Carbs:** 2.4g | **Fiber:** 0.7g | **Erythritol:** 16g

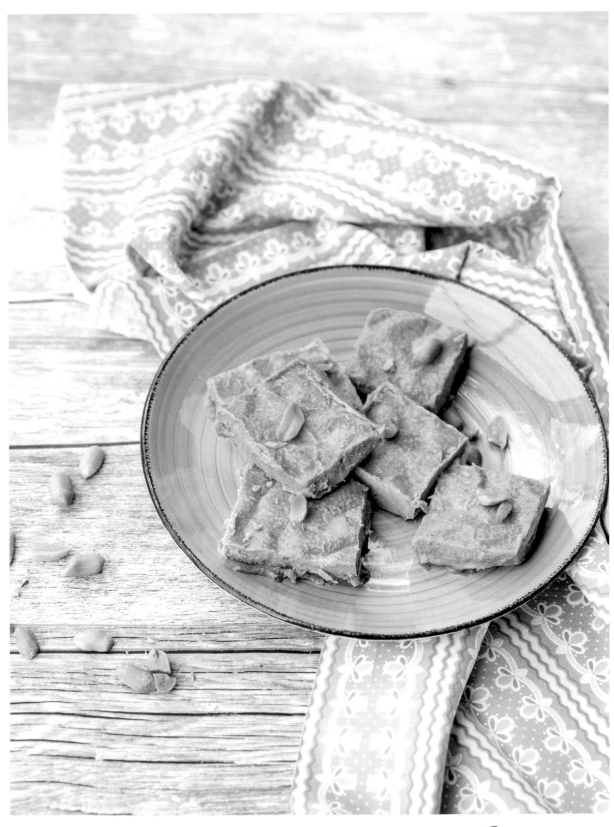

# KRISTIE'S SOUTHERN-STYLE PIMENTO CHEESE

**MAKES** 8 servings | **PREP TIME:** 8 minutes, plus 1 hour to chill (not including time to cook bacon if not purchased precooked)

*My best friend's mom made the best pimento cheese I ever tasted. Ever. Her pimento cheese was far better than my recipe. It might be because of the cheese, but I suspect it's the extra love she stirred into it. She usually made it at the request of others, and we sure did request it often! Her recipe didn't use cream cheese, but I like to include it for the creamy texture. Of course, we always ate pimento cheese in a sandwich or on crackers, but what we missed is how good this stuff is on its own, eaten with a spoon! I love to put a hefty dollop on a burger or any type of meat. I also enjoy eating it with deli meat, cucumber chips, celery sticks, sliced pepperoni, or pork rinds.*

**1 cup mayonnaise**

**2 ounces cream cheese (¼ cup), softened**

**8 ounces sharp cheddar cheese, shredded (about 2 cups)**

**8 ounces mild cheddar cheese, shredded (about 2 cups)**

**⅓ cup cooked bacon pieces**

**3 tablespoons jarred diced pimentos**

**1 tablespoon Worcestershire sauce**

**¼ teaspoon garlic powder**

**¼ teaspoon cayenne pepper (optional)**

**Sliced jalapeño peppers, for garnish (optional)**

In a large bowl, mix together the mayonnaise and cream cheese until well blended. Add the shredded cheeses and stir well. Add the bacon, pimentos, Worcestershire sauce, garlic powder, and cayenne pepper, if using, and stir until thoroughly combined. Refrigerate for at least 1 hour before serving. Garnish with sliced jalapeños, if desired. Store leftovers in the refrigerator for up to 1 week.

**Variation: Baked Pimento Cheese.** Pimento cheese is also delicious as a warm dip served with crudités, pork rinds, pepperoni chips, or cheese chips. To make Baked Pimento Cheese, preheat the oven to 350°F. Spread the prepared pimento cheese in a shallow 1½-quart baking dish. Bake, uncovered, for 20 to 25 minutes, or until the cheese is melted and bubbly and lightly browned on top. Serve warm. Store leftovers in the refrigerator for up to 3 days.

Calories: 449 | Fat: 36.1g | Protein: 19.8g | Carbs: 4.2g | Fiber: 0.8g

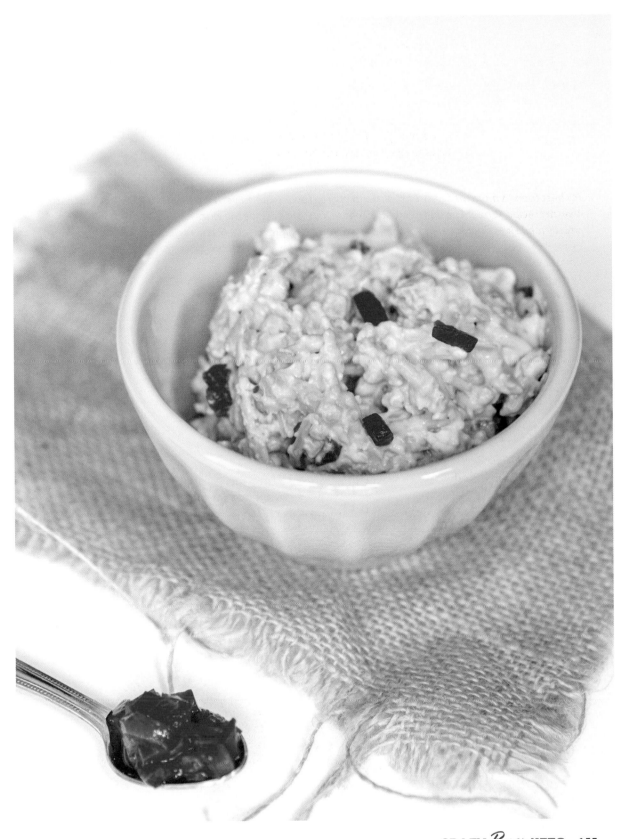

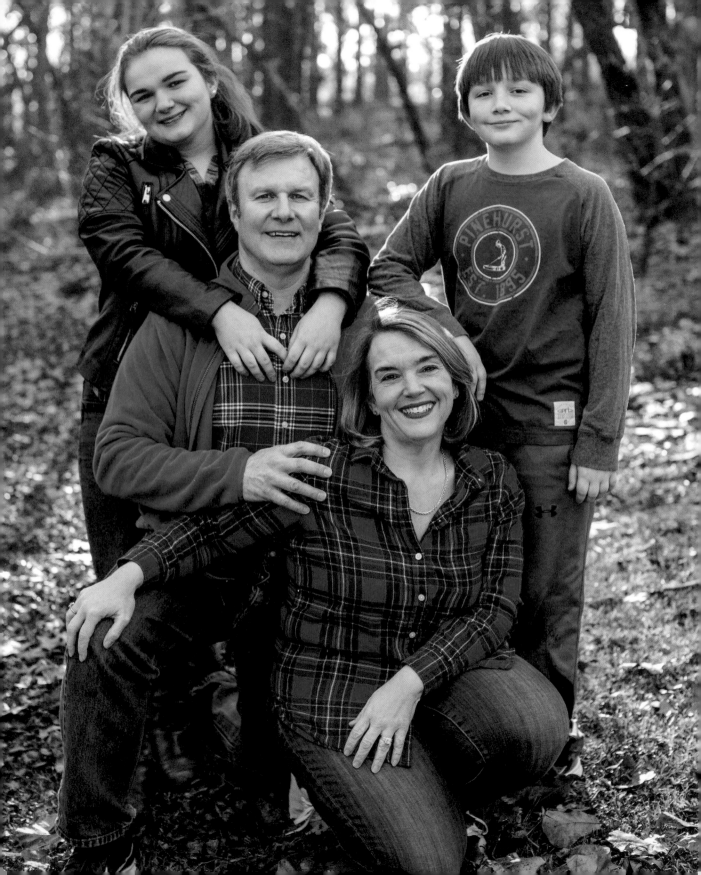

# ACKNOWLEDGMENTS

As always, I'm grateful for the love and support of my family, who bravely taste-test every recipe at least once, but often much more, bravely telling me whether it's a keeper or to "keep trying." Their honesty makes my recipes better.

My immense gratitude to the great folks at Victory Belt—Pam, the editor with enormous patience; Holly, who doesn't miss a detail; Susan, who helps share the best of my books; Justin, who is such a talented designer that I always look forward to seeing his magic in print; Lance, who keeps all of the pieces moving; and Erich, whose vision has us all here working together! Thank you to each of you for your work and collaboration. It's a wonderful reminder that all of us working together with our respective strengths create something far bigger than any of us could alone.

Special thanks to the volunteer moderators who are online around the clock throughout different time zones helping me help others who are just as desperate as I once was find a way to lose weight and improve their health. Your work is invaluable. We are changing lives together, one family at a time. Thank you for your unselfish love and support for our members and for me and my family.

To my followers, thank you for believing in me enough to buy my books, try the recipes, and keep sharing your own success stories. It's the only way we're ever going to make a difference in the health of our loved ones and in our communities.

Lastly, this book would not have come together without the help of my sweet friends Mary Bridschge and Jenny Lowder. Thank you for the marathon food photo days. With Mary in the kitchen cooking and cleaning and Jenny behind the lens, there's nothing we can't do! You helped me power through the brown foods yet again. Thank you!

# Shopping GUIDE

As I've searched for convenient options, I've found that ingredient quality and carb counts vary widely, so I thought it might be helpful to provide you with a list of the brands that I prefer to use. While availability may vary by region or country, these are brands that I seek out when I'm shopping for convenience products. Please note that manufacturers sometimes change the ingredients in their products, which may affect the nutritional information.

As a general rule, look for the brands that have the fewest ingredients and that do not contain added sugar, fructose, high-fructose corn syrup, molasses, honey, cornstarch, dextrose, or maltodextrin.

## MEATS AND CHEESES

**Bacon (precooked)**—The precooked bacon that I use most often comes from warehouse stores, such as Kirkland brand from Costco and Hormel brand from Sam's Club. Aldi has precooked bacon in smaller packages that are perfect for travel because they don't need to be refrigerated until opened. Those smaller packages contain five to seven slices each, which generally can be consumed in one meal.

**Canned meats**—With regard to the types of canned meats mentioned in this book, brands vary a good deal. Even within the same brand, the ingredients vary. For that reason, I always look at the ingredients first. Many canned meats are packed in water, which is ideal because I can add any desired fats. Tuna is likely to be packed in oil. In that case, I select tuna packed in olive oil over canola oil.

**Cheese**—Look for cheeses that are made from milk and do not contain added vegetable oils.

**Deli meats**—Boar's Head, Dietz & Watson, and Hormel Naturals are brands without a lot of fillers or sweeteners. Ingredients vary by type of meat, but ingredient lists are often available online. Roast beef is less likely to have added sugars than ham or turkey.

**Jerky**—Chomps, Nick's Sticks, and Organic Valley brands are the least likely to contain food starches or sugars. In addition to checking the ingredient lists, always check the nutrition labels. Any jerky with less than 2 grams of carbs per serving is generally safe. Unfortunately, I've seen jerky with carbs as high as 8 to 12 grams per serving.

**Mexican chorizo**—Be sure to read the labels to avoid added wheat and grains. I often use the Supremo brand, which is available at most national grocers. La Banderita brand is also very good but may be more difficult to find.

**Parmesan cheese**—Never buy canned Parmesan cheese, even if it's refrigerated! Real Parmesan does not have the texture of fine sawdust. Real Parmesan is sold shredded, shaved, or in chunks.

# SAUCES

**Béarnaise**—Although I don't call for béarnaise sauce in any of the recipes in this book, it's one of my favorite keto sauces. It adds yummy fat and flavor to any meal, and it is quick and easy to use when you buy a commercial premade sauce. I've found only one shelf-stable brand of béarnaise, and it's made by Christian Potier. While it isn't the same as homemade, it is a great option for adding fat and flavor to a simple meal like a Pan-Seared Steak (page 94).

**Blue cheese dressing**—Another good fatty "sauce" to keep on hand, blue cheese dressing can be used to top a salad dressing or as a dip for meats. Look in the refrigerated section of the grocery store for the product with the fewest food starches and sugars added. Marie's is often a good brand.

**Buffalo wing sauce**—Frank's RedHot is the brand I use most frequently, and it is generally reliable for taste and ingredients.

**Chimichurri**—I don't call for chimichurri in any of the recipes in this book, but I often turn to it to add excitement to my keto meals. A thick herb sauce that's Argentinian in origin, chimichurri is excellent over steak or any other grilled or roasted meat. Badia makes a very good chimichurri with an olive oil base.

**Enchilada sauce**—Many popular brands contain food starches and industrial seed oils. El Pato, Las Palmas, and Rosarita do not contain food starches but may contain small amounts of canola oil or cottonseed oil, which makes them preferable to brands that contain starches or sugar.

**Hollandaise**—Christian Potier makes a very good shelf-stable hollandaise that can be served over meats or vegetables. The ingredients are great and the carbs minimal. Even though hollandaise is easy to make, it's worth mentioning this convenient alternative, particularly if you're traveling or need something super fast.

**Marinara sauce**—Rao's is a great low-carb brand, but it can be a bit pricey and hard to find. If you can't track down Rao's, compare the nutrition information for the brands you do find, and stick to those that have fewer than 6 grams of carbs per ½-cup serving.

**Mayonnaise**—Many commercial mayonnaises are made with soybean oil or canola oil and contain added sugar, which I tend to avoid. My preference is the Primal Kitchen brand, which is made with avocado oil. The rest of my family is steadfastly devoted to Duke's brand mayonnaise, which has no sugar but is made with canola oil. Because they use mayonnaise minimally, taste is their guide, and Duke's wins out.

**Pesto**—Unlike other brands, Mezzetta basil pesto does not contain food starches or seed oils. It's my preferred brand for taste and ingredients.

**Ranch dressing**—Hidden Valley Classic Ranch is my family's favorite bottled dressing, even though I prefer to make my own ranch dressing. Be sure to buy the full-fat version, as the reduced-fat one has more carbs because of added sugars and food starches.

**Salsa**—Jack's Special Salsa Mild has great ingredients and only 1 gram of carbs per tablespoon. You can find it in the refrigerated produce section of most grocery stores. For a shelf-stable option, Pace Chunky Salsa Mild has 3 grams of carbs per 2-tablespoon serving, and the ingredients are good.

**Tomato sauce**—Compare labels and look for tomato sauce without sugar in the ingredient list. Often, store brands have the fewest ingredients and the least carbs.

# OTHER

**Almond butter**—Look for brands that contain only almonds and salt. Almond butter is very thick, and most brands need to be stirred well before use.

**Bone broth powdered drink mix**—Made by Ketologie, this drink mix is my preferred option for bouillon in my cooking. It is made with excellent ingredients and has a great taste. It comes in multiple flavors. For the recipes in this book, I use the roast chicken flavor. It is available only on the Ketologie website or from Amazon. If you can find a good-quality chicken bouillon made with keto-friendly ingredients, feel free to use that in the recipes that call for powdered chicken bone broth.

**Chicken broth**—If you don't have time to make your own broth, try the Imagine brand. It is made with very good ingredients. When comparing brands, look specifically at the carb counts per serving and select the product with the least carbs.

**Chipotle peppers**—My preferred brand is Pueblo Lindo, which has 1 gram of carbs per ounce. Unlike other brands, the ingredients do not include food starches, soybean oil, or canola oil.

**Corn extract**—I've never found this product in stores, but it is available online. Amoretti is an expensive brand, but it's the best I've found for flavor and ingredients. A small bottle lasts a long time.

**Cream**—Trader Joe's sells a shelf-stable whipping cream that is also available on Amazon in case you don't have a store nearby. It's a great Plan B item and useful for travel since it does not require refrigeration until opened. It can be used in any recipe in this book that calls for heavy cream.

**Diced tomatoes and green chilies**—Like all tomato products, be sure to check the ingredients for added sugars. Casa Mamita and Rotel are generally lower in carbs than other brands.

**Egg white protein powder**—If you need to use egg white protein powder to avoid the dairy in whey protein isolate, Jay Robb is a good brand to buy.

**Ghee**—Ghee is simply clarified butter that's been simmered longer, until all of the moisture evaporates and the milk solids begin to brown, resulting in a fat with a slightly nutty flavor and a relatively high smoke point. Because nearly all of the casein and lactose have been removed from ghee, it is typically safe to consume for people who avoid dairy unless they are extremely sensitive to dairy. Trader Joe's offers an inexpensive option, as do many common grocers.

I've found ghee travel packets from only one company, and that is 4th & Heart. The packet has a convenient tab for easy opening. There are two flavors, original and vanilla. The original flavor can be drizzled over vegetables or meats to add fat. The vanilla flavor is excellent for adding to coffee.

**Parmesan cheese crisps**—For this book, I used the Whisps brand of cheese crisps. They are made with 100 percent cheese and are the perfect size for making cheese cracker snacks (see page 138). Be sure to choose a brand that contains only cheese and perhaps some natural seasonings or flavorings. There are commercial "cheese" crackers that include wheat and/or starches or other fillers; avoid those!

**Peanut butter**—All you need is peanuts and salt. If there's anything else in the ingredient list, put the jar back on the shelf and leave it there! Crazy Richard's and Trader Joe's are the two brands most frequently stocked in my cabinets.

**Pork rinds**—My favorite pork rinds are the big, fluffy original flavor from Carolina Country Snacks. While there are pork cracklin's, those tend to be very hard and thin and are not ideal for the recipes in this book. Some brands have more fat and taste more like pork than others. In addition to Carolina Country Snacks, I like the Turkey Creek brand, which is often sold at dollar stores, and the Epic brand, which is one of the few that offer seasoned pork rinds without food starches or sugars.

**Psyllium fiber**—The only drawback to using psyllium fiber is that it can turn baked goods purple. Source Naturals and Now Foods are the two brands least likely to have this effect. Besides those, most brands are just ground psyllium husks and should work well.

**Salt**—I tend to use Redmond Real Salt, which is a fine-grained sea salt, although some people see an advantage in using an iodized table salt.

**Whey protein isolate (unflavored)**—My preferred brands are Isopure and Jay Robb because they do not contain added sweeteners and because they have zero carbs. See page 13 for a discussion of the use of this ingredient in the recipes in this book.

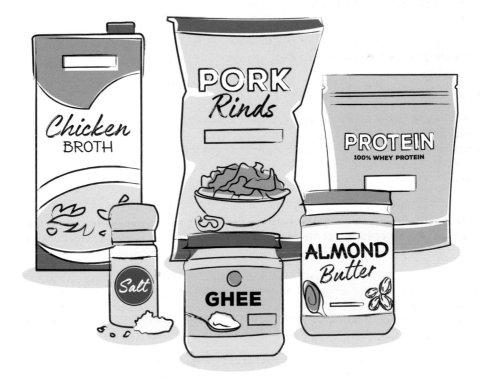

# PREP AND ALLERGEN INDEX

| RECIPE | PAGE | 🍳 | 〰️ | 🍲 | 15 | 30 | 🥛 | 🥚 |
|---|---|---|---|---|---|---|---|---|
| Good Morning Granola | 30 | | | ✓ | | | O | |
| Lemon Minute Muffins | 32 | | ✓ | | ✓ | | O | |
| Loco Mocha Muffins | 34 | | | ✓ | | ✓ | | |
| Everything Bagels | 36 | | | ✓ | | ✓ | | ✓ |
| Salad Bar Crustless Quiche | 38 | | | ✓ | | | | ✓ |
| 2-Minute Microwave Omelet | 40 | | ✓ | | ✓ | | O | ✓ |
| Crazy Busy Waffles | 42 | | | ✓ | | ✓ | | |
| Simple Pancake Syrup | 42 | | | ✓ | ✓ | | O | ✓ |
| Buffalo Chicken Ranch No-tato Salad | 50 | | ✓ | | ✓ | | | ✓ |
| Double Bacon Cheeseburger Bake | 52 | | | ✓ | | | | ✓ |
| 5-Minute Lasagna | 54 | | ✓ | ✓ | ✓ | | | ✓ |
| Individual BBQ Chicken Pizzas | 56 | | | ✓ | | ✓ | | |
| Buffalo Chicken Bake with Bacon and Ranch | 58 | | | ✓ | | | | ✓ |
| Nachos Two Ways | 60 | | | | | ✓ | | ✓ |
| Chicken à la King | 62 | | | ✓ | | ✓ | | ✓ |
| Chile Rellenos Casserole | 64 | | | ✓ | | | | ✓ |
| Baked Chicken Parmesan | 66 | | | | | | | ✓ |
| Chipotle Chicken Salad | 68 | ✓ | | ✓ | ✓ | | ✓ | ✓ |
| Chili-Lime Wings | 70 | | | | | | ✓ | ✓ |
| Greek Wings | 72 | | | | | | O | ✓ |
| Traditional Buffalo Wings | 73 | | | | | | O | ✓ |
| Cold Tossed Pizza Bowl | 74 | ✓ | | | ✓ | | | ✓ |
| Deconstructed Chicken Cordon Bleu | 76 | | | ✓ | | | | ✓ |
| Easy Chicken and Beef Enchilada Bake | 78 | | | ✓ | | | | ✓ |
| One-Pan Chicken Alfredo with Spaghetti Squash | 80 | | | | | ✓ | | ✓ |
| Shrimp Salad–Stuffed Avocado Boats | 82 | ✓ | | | ✓ | | | ✓ |
| Thai Chicken Slaw with Peanut Sauce | 84 | ✓ | | | ✓ | | ✓ | |
| Fried Salmon Patties | 86 | | | | ✓ | | O | ✓ |

| RECIPE | PAGE | | | | 15 | 30 | | |
|---|---|---|---|---|---|---|---|---|
| Greek Meatballs | 88 | | | ✓ | | ✓ | | ✓ |
| Quick Chicken Chowder | 90 | | | ✓ | | ✓ | | ✓ |
| Easy Egg and Bacon Salad | 92 | ✓ | | | ✓ | | | ✓ |
| Pan-Seared Steak | 94 | | | | ✓ | | ✓ | ✓ |
| Salad Bar Stir-Fry | 96 | | | | ✓ | | ✓ | ✓ |
| Lazy Slow Cooker Beef Stew | 98 | | | ✓ | | | | ✓ |
| Spicy Poppin' Shrimp | 100 | | | | ✓ | | O | ✓ |
| Egg Drop Soup | 102 | | ✓ | | ✓ | | ✓ | ✓ |
| One-Bowl Creamed Spinach and Artichokes | 110 | | ✓ | | ✓ | | | ✓ |
| Simple Wedge Salad | 112 | ✓ | | | ✓ | | | ✓ |
| Pan-Fried Cauliflower with Pesto | 114 | | | | ✓ | | | |
| Speedy Creamed Spinach | 116 | | | | ✓ | | | ✓ |
| Unstuffed Jalapeño Popper Casserole | 118 | | | | | ✓ | | ✓ |
| Creamy Cucumber and Red Onion Salad | 120 | ✓ | | | ✓ | | | ✓ |
| Microwaved Spaghetti Squash | 122 | | ✓ | ✓ | ✓ | | O | ✓ |
| Mexican Fiesta Cauli Rice | 124 | | | | ✓ | | O | ✓ |
| Loaded Baked Yellow Squash | 126 | | ✓ | | ✓ | | | ✓ |
| Creamy Avocado Salsa | 128 | ✓ | | | ✓ | | | ✓ |
| Feta Cream Sauce | 130 | ✓ | | | ✓ | | | ✓ |
| Tzatziki Sauce | 132 | ✓ | | | ✓ | | | ✓ |
| Thai Peanut Sauce | 134 | | ✓ | | ✓ | | ✓ | |
| Strawberry Cream Pie | 142 | | | ✓ | ✓ | | | |
| Cheesecake in Minutes | 144 | | ✓ | ✓ | ✓ | | | |
| Chili-Lime Trail Mix | 146 | | | ✓ | | | | |
| Forgotten Cookies | 148 | | | ✓ | | | ✓ | O |
| Whipped Cheesecake Dream | 150 | ✓ | | | ✓ | | | ✓ |
| Peanut Butter Fudge | 152 | | | ✓ | ✓ | | | |
| Kristie's Southern-Style Pimento Cheese | 154 | ✓ | | | ✓ | | | ✓ |

# RECIPE INDEX

## BREAKFASTS

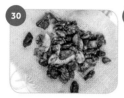
**30**
Good Morning Granola

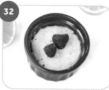
**32**
Lemon Minute Muffins

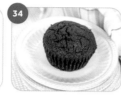
**34**
Loco Mocha Muffins

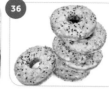
**36**
Everything Bagels

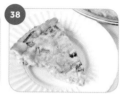
**38**
Salad Bar Crustless Quiche

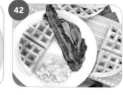
**40**
2-Minute Microwave Omelet

**42**
Crazy Busy Waffles

## MAINS

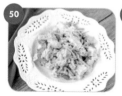
**50**
Buffalo Chicken Ranch No-tato Salad

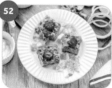
**52**
Double Bacon Cheeseburger Bake

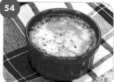
**54**
5-Minute Lasagna

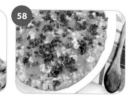
**56**
Individual BBQ Chicken Pizzas

**58**
Buffalo Chicken Bake with Bacon and Ranch

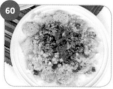
**60**
Nachos Two Ways

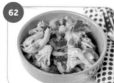
**62**
Chicken à la King

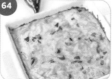
**64**
Chile Rellenos Casserole

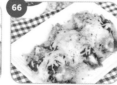
**66**
Baked Chicken Parmesan

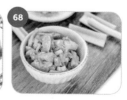
**68**
Chipotle Chicken Salad

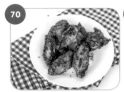
**70**
Chili-Lime Wings

**72**
Greek Wings

**73**
Traditional Buffalo Wings

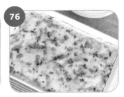
**74**
Cold Tossed Pizza Bowl

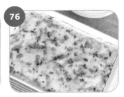
**76**
Deconstructed Chicken Cordon Bleu

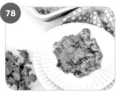
**78**
Easy Chicken and Beef Enchilada Bake

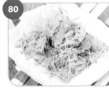
**80**
One-Pan Chicken Alfredo with Spaghetti Squash

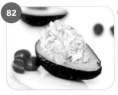
**82**
Shrimp Salad–Stuffed Avocado Boats

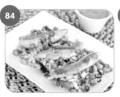
**84**
Thai Chicken Slaw with Peanut Sauce

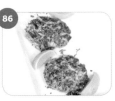
**86**
Fried Salmon Patties

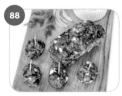
**88**
Greek Meatballs

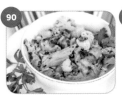
**90**
Quick Chicken Chowder

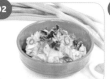
**92**
Easy Egg and Bacon Salad

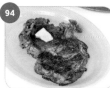
**94**
Pan-Seared Steak

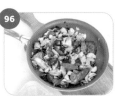
**96**
Salad Bar Stir-Fry

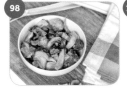
**98**
Lazy Slow Cooker Beef Stew

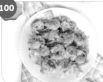
**100**
Spicy Poppin' Shrimp

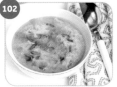
**102**
Egg Drop Soup

## SIDES & SAUCES

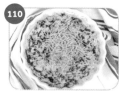
**110**
One-Bowl Creamed Spinach and Artichokes

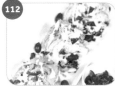
**112**
Simple Wedge Salad

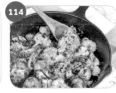
**114**
Pan-Fried Cauliflower with Pesto

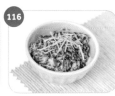
**116**
Speedy Creamed Spinach

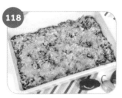
**118**
Unstuffed Jalapeño Popper Casserole

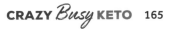

## SIDES & SAUCES *(continued)*

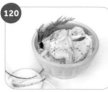
**120**
Creamy Cucumber
and Red Onion Salad

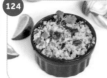
**122**
Microwaved
Spaghetti Squash

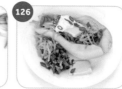
**124**
Mexican Fiesta
Cauli Rice

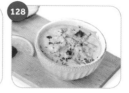
**126**
Loaded Baked
Yellow Squash

**128**
Creamy Avocado
Salsa

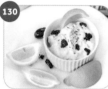
**130**
Feta Cream Sauce

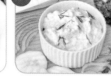
**132**
Tzatziki Sauce

**134**
Thai Peanut Sauce

## TREATS & SNACKS

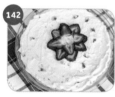
**142**
Strawberry
Cream Pie

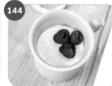
**144**
Cheesecake in
Minutes

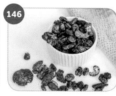
**146**
Chili-Lime Trail Mix

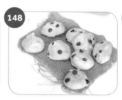
**148**
Forgotten Cookies

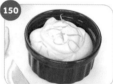
**150**
Whipped
Cheesecake Dream

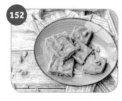
**152**
Peanut Butter Fudge

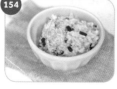
**154**
Kristie's
Southern-Style
Pimento Cheese

# GENERAL INDEX

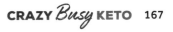

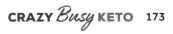

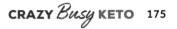

# ABOUT THE AUTHOR

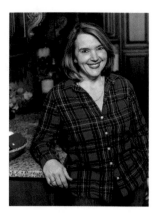

Kristie Sullivan spent most of her life being obese. In June 2013, she found keto, lost over 100 pounds, and has been keto ever since, even when crazy busy! She is the author of *Journey to Health: A Journey Worth Taking, Keto Living Day by Day,* and *Keto Gatherings.* After retiring early from a career in higher education assessment, evaluation, research, and accreditation, she has dedicated her life's work to showing others that the ketogenic lifestyle is not only practical, but truly sustainable for a lifetime. You can find her on YouTube (Cooking Keto with Kristie), on Facebook (on her public page, Simply Keto with Kristie Sullivan, and in her closed group, Low Carb Journey to Health: Cooking Keto with Kristie), and on her website, cookingketowithkristie. com.

Kristie also serves as Head of Community for Diet Doctor, a website centered around low-carb and ketogenic diets, where she has her own cooking show and provides seasonal recipes. She lives in the beautiful Sandhills region of North Carolina with her husband, David, and their two children, Grace and Jonathan, who are growing up keto.